CONTENTS

Chapter 1: Introduction to Cough-Variant Asthma 1
Chapter 2: Pathophysiology of Cough-Variant Asthma 15
Chapter 3: Trigger Factors and Environmental Influences 40
Chapter 4: Clinical Evaluation and Diagnostic Approach 69
Chapter 5: Management and Treatment Strategies 97
Chapter 6: Complications and Comorbidities 115
Chapter 7: Advances in Research and Future Directions 146
Chapter 8: Holistic Approach to Cough-Variant Asthma Management 173

CHAPTER 1: INTRODUCTION TO COUGH-VARIANT ASTHMA

Definition and Overview of Cough-Variant Asthma

Cough-variant asthma (CVA) stands as a unique clinical entity within the spectrum of asthma, characterized predominantly by a chronic, non-productive cough as the sole or predominant symptom. Unlike classic asthma, where wheezing and shortness of breath are prominent features, cough-variant asthma may present challenges in diagnosis due to the absence of these hallmark symptoms. Nevertheless, it shares the underlying pathophysiological mechanisms with typical asthma, primarily involving airway inflammation and hyperresponsiveness.

The defining feature of CVA is the persistent cough, often triggered or exacerbated by various factors such as allergens, respiratory infections, environmental pollutants, exercise, or emotional stress. This cough typically persists for more than 8 weeks and may worsen at night or upon exposure to triggers. Patients with CVA may experience occasional episodes of dyspnea or wheezing, particularly during exacerbations or when the disease progresses to involve other components of the airway.

It is essential to recognize cough-variant asthma as a distinct clinical phenotype, as its management and treatment strategies may differ from those of classic asthma. While both conditions share common pharmacological interventions such as inhaled corticosteroids and bronchodilators, the emphasis in CVA management often lies in targeting the cough reflex and airway inflammation specifically.

The pathophysiology of cough-variant asthma mirrors that of classic asthma, characterized by chronic inflammation of the airways, bronchial hyperresponsiveness, and airway remodeling. Immunological mechanisms play a central role, involving the activation of various immune cells such as mast cells, eosinophils, and T-helper cells, particularly the Th2 subset. These cells release inflammatory mediators such as histamine, leukotrienes, and cytokines, leading to bronchoconstriction, mucus hypersecretion, and airway edema.

One key aspect distinguishing CVA from other causes of chronic cough is the presence of airway hyperresponsiveness, which refers to an exaggerated bronchoconstrictor response to various stimuli. This hyperreactivity contributes to the persistence and severity of cough episodes in patients with CVA, even in the absence of overt airflow limitation or wheezing.

Diagnosing cough-variant asthma requires a thorough clinical evaluation, including a detailed patient history, physical examination, and appropriate diagnostic tests. Given the absence of wheezing or dyspnea in many cases, clinicians must maintain a high index of suspicion for CVA, particularly in patients with a history of allergic rhinitis, atopy, or other allergic conditions.

Pulmonary function tests, including spirometry and bronchial provocation tests, play a crucial role in confirming the diagnosis of CVA. Spirometry may reveal normal baseline lung function but can demonstrate reversible airflow obstruction following bronchodilator administration. Bronchial provocation tests, such as the methacholine challenge test, help assess airway hyperresponsiveness by measuring the degree of bronchoconstriction in response to a bronchoconstrictor agent.

Additional diagnostic modalities, including exhaled nitric oxide measurement, allergy testing, and chest imaging, may be employed to further characterize the underlying inflammation and identify potential triggers or comorbid conditions contributing to cough-variant asthma.

In summary, cough-variant asthma represents a distinct phenotype of asthma characterized by chronic cough as the primary symptom. While its diagnosis may pose challenges due to the absence of typical asthma features, a comprehensive evaluation incorporating clinical assessment and objective testing is essential for accurate diagnosis and appropriate management. Recognizing the pathophysiological mechanisms underlying CVA and tailoring treatment strategies accordingly are crucial steps in optimizing outcomes for patients with this condition.

Prevalence and Incidence Rates of Cough-Variant Asthma

Understanding the prevalence and incidence rates of cough-variant asthma (CVA) is essential for recognizing the burden of this condition on public health and healthcare systems, as well as for guiding clinical practice and resource allocation. While cough-variant asthma shares common pathophysiological mechanisms with classic asthma, its unique clinical presentation and diagnostic challenges warrant specific attention to epidemiological data.

Prevalence of Cough-Variant Asthma:

Estimating the prevalence of CVA presents inherent challenges due to variations in study methodologies, diagnostic criteria, and population demographics. Nonetheless, research indicates that CVA represents a significant proportion of asthma cases, particularly among patients with chronic cough. Studies have reported prevalence rates ranging from 20% to 40% among individuals presenting with chronic cough, making it one of the most common causes of chronic cough in both pediatric and adult populations.

Population-based studies further support the substantial prevalence of CVA, highlighting its significance as a clinical entity. While classic asthma remains the predominant form of the disease, accounting for the majority of asthma cases, CVA represents a notable subset, particularly among patients with atopic conditions such as allergic rhinitis or eczema.

Moreover, the prevalence of CVA appears to vary across different age groups and demographic profiles. While pediatric studies have reported a higher prevalence of CVA among children with chronic cough, adult populations, especially those with late-onset asthma or atopic predispositions, also demonstrate a considerable burden of this condition. Additionally, geographical factors, environmental exposures, and socioeconomic determinants may influence the prevalence of CVA within specific populations or regions.

Incidence Rates of Cough-Variant Asthma:

Assessing the incidence rates of CVA poses challenges due to limited longitudinal data and variability in diagnostic practices over time. Unlike prevalence, which reflects the proportion of existing cases within a population, incidence measures the rate of new cases emerging over a specific period.

Longitudinal studies tracking individuals at risk for asthma development have provided insights into the incidence rates of CVA among susceptible populations. These studies often involve cohorts of children or adults with a history of allergic rhinitis, atopy, or other allergic conditions, who are followed prospectively to identify new-onset asthma cases, including CVA.

While precise incidence rates of CVA remain elusive, emerging evidence suggests that this phenotype may account for a considerable proportion of incident asthma cases, particularly among individuals with allergic predispositions or a history of recurrent respiratory infections. The transition from acute respiratory symptoms, such as cough or wheezing associated with viral infections, to persistent cough-variant asthma highlights the dynamic nature of disease progression and the importance of early recognition and intervention.

Furthermore, environmental factors, including exposure to allergens, pollutants, or occupational hazards, may influence the incidence of CVA within specific populations or occupational groups. Occupational asthma, characterized by work-related respiratory symptoms, including cough, may manifest as cough-variant asthma in susceptible individuals exposed to occupational allergens or irritants.

Conclusion:

In conclusion, cough-variant asthma represents a significant clinical phenotype within the spectrum of asthma, characterized by chronic cough as the predominant symptom. While precise estimates of prevalence and incidence rates may vary across studies and populations, evidence suggests that CVA contributes substantially to the overall burden of asthma, particularly among individuals with allergic predispositions or chronic respiratory symptoms.

Continued efforts to improve diagnostic accuracy, enhance epidemiological surveillance, and implement targeted interventions are essential for effectively addressing the challenges posed by cough-variant asthma and reducing its impact on individual patients and public health systems. By raising awareness, promoting early detection, and optimizing management strategies, healthcare providers can better serve the needs of patients with cough-variant asthma and improve their quality of life.

Clinical Presentation and Symptoms of Cough-Variant Asthma

Cough-variant asthma (CVA) presents a unique challenge in clinical practice due to its atypical symptoms and subtle manifestations. Unlike classic asthma, where wheezing and dyspnea are prominent features, CVA primarily manifests as a chronic, non-productive cough. Understanding the clinical presentation and symptoms of CVA is crucial for accurate diagnosis and appropriate management.

Characteristics of Cough-Variant Asthma:

The hallmark feature of CVA is a persistent cough, lasting for more than 8 weeks, which may be the sole or predominant symptom in affected individuals. This cough often occurs without associated wheezing or dyspnea, making it difficult to recognize as a manifestation of asthma. Patients may describe the cough as dry, hacking, or paroxysmal, with exacerbations triggered by various factors such as allergens, respiratory infections, exercise, or emotional stress.

The timing and pattern of cough episodes can provide valuable clues to differentiate CVA from other causes of chronic cough. Patients with CVA may experience worsening of cough at night, upon awakening, or upon exposure to specific triggers, such as cold air, strong odors, or environmental pollutants. The absence of cough during sleep or physical exertion may further distinguish CVA from other respiratory conditions, such as gastroesophageal reflux disease (GERD) or upper airway cough syndrome (formerly known as postnasal drip syndrome).

In some cases, patients with CVA may develop additional symptoms beyond cough, particularly during exacerbations or when the disease progresses to involve other components of the airway. These symptoms may include wheezing, chest tightness, shortness of breath, or nocturnal awakenings due to respiratory symptoms. However, these features are often less pronounced compared to classic asthma and may not be present in all cases of CVA.

Clinical Evaluation and Differential Diagnosis:

Diagnosing CVA requires a comprehensive clinical evaluation, including a detailed patient history, physical examination, and appropriate diagnostic tests. Clinicians should inquire about the duration, frequency, and characteristics of the cough, as well as any associated symptoms or triggers. A thorough assessment of past medical history, including allergic conditions, respiratory infections, or environmental exposures, is essential to identify potential risk factors for CVA.

Physical examination findings in patients with CVA may be unremarkable or may reveal subtle signs of airway inflammation, such as mild wheezing or prolonged expiration. However, the absence of these findings does not exclude the diagnosis of CVA, as cough may be the only presenting symptom in some cases.

Differential diagnosis of chronic cough encompasses a broad range of conditions, including but not limited to asthma, GERD, upper airway cough syndrome, eosinophilic bronchitis, bronchiectasis, or medication-induced cough. Distinguishing CVA from these conditions requires careful consideration of clinical features, diagnostic test results, and response to therapeutic interventions.

Impact on Quality of Life:

The chronic nature of cough-variant asthma can significantly impact patients' quality of life, leading to physical discomfort, social embarrassment, and psychological distress. The persistent cough may interfere with daily activities, such as work, school, or sleep, resulting in fatigue, irritability, or impaired concentration.

Furthermore, the insidious onset and subtle nature of CVA symptoms may delay diagnosis and initiation of appropriate treatment, exacerbating the burden of disease on affected individuals. Patients may undergo multiple diagnostic evaluations or receive ineffective therapies for presumed causes of cough before achieving a correct diagnosis of CVA.

Conclusion:

In conclusion, cough-variant asthma presents a unique clinical phenotype characterized by a chronic, non-productive cough as the predominant symptom. Recognizing the subtle manifestations of CVA, understanding its impact on patients' quality of life, and differentiating it from other causes of chronic cough are essential steps in providing optimal care for affected individuals. By raising awareness, promoting early diagnosis, and implementing evidence-based management strategies, healthcare providers can effectively address the challenges posed by cough-variant asthma and improve outcomes for patients.

Differential Diagnosis of Cough-Variant Asthma

Diagnosing cough-variant asthma (CVA) requires careful consideration of the clinical presentation, diagnostic test results, and exclusion of other potential causes of chronic cough. The differential diagnosis of CVA encompasses a broad range of conditions, including respiratory and non-respiratory disorders, each with distinct pathophysiological mechanisms and management approaches. By understanding the key features of these conditions and employing a systematic diagnostic approach, clinicians can accurately identify and appropriately manage patients with CVA.

1. Classic Asthma:

Classic asthma represents the prototypical form of the disease, characterized by episodic wheezing, dyspnea, chest tightness, and cough. Unlike CVA, where cough is the predominant symptom, classic asthma typically presents with a combination of respiratory symptoms, often triggered by allergens, exercise, cold air, or respiratory infections. The presence of wheezing, reversible airflow obstruction on pulmonary function tests, and positive response to bronchodilators supports the diagnosis of classic asthma.

2. Gastroesophageal Reflux Disease (GERD):

GERD is a common gastrointestinal disorder characterized by retrograde flow of gastric contents into the esophagus, leading to symptoms such as heartburn, regurgitation, and chronic cough. Chronic cough associated with GERD often occurs in the absence of other respiratory symptoms and may worsen upon lying down or after meals. Diagnostic evaluation typically includes esophageal pH monitoring or impedance testing to assess for reflux events, as well as response to acid-suppressive therapy.

3. Upper Airway Cough Syndrome (UACS):

Formerly known as postnasal drip syndrome, UACS refers to a condition characterized by excessive mucus production and irritation of the upper airway, leading to chronic cough. Common causes include allergic rhinitis, sinusitis, or nasal polyps. Patients with UACS may experience nasal congestion, throat clearing, or a sensation of mucus dripping down the back of the throat. Diagnosis involves clinical evaluation, nasal endoscopy, and imaging studies to identify underlying sinonasal pathology.

4. Eosinophilic Bronchitis:

Eosinophilic bronchitis shares similarities with asthma, including airway inflammation and eosinophilic infiltration, but lacks the characteristic features of airflow limitation or bronchial hyperresponsiveness. Patients with eosinophilic bronchitis present with chronic cough and sputum eosinophilia, often without evidence of variable airflow obstruction or atopy. Diagnosis requires sputum analysis to confirm eosinophilic inflammation and exclusion of other causes of chronic cough.

5. Bronchiectasis:

Bronchiectasis is a chronic respiratory condition characterized by irreversible dilation and thickening of the bronchial walls, leading to recurrent respiratory infections, chronic cough, and sputum production. Unlike CVA, which primarily presents with cough as the predominant symptom, bronchiectasis often manifests with purulent sputum, hemoptysis, and recurrent pulmonary exacerbations. High-resolution chest computed tomography (HRCT) is the gold standard for diagnosing bronchiectasis and assessing the extent of bronchial damage.

6. Medication-Induced Cough:

Certain medications, such as angiotensin-converting enzyme (ACE) inhibitors, beta-blockers, or nonsteroidal anti-inflammatory drugs (NSAIDs), can induce chronic cough as a side effect. ACE inhibitor-induced cough is particularly well-recognized and often presents with dry, persistent cough within weeks to months of starting the medication. Discontinuation of the offending agent typically resolves the cough, confirming the diagnosis of medication-induced cough.

7. Chronic Obstructive Pulmonary Disease (COPD):

COPD is a progressive respiratory condition characterized by airflow limitation, typically associated with a history of smoking and exposure to environmental pollutants. While chronic cough is a common feature of COPD, it is often accompanied by other respiratory symptoms such as dyspnea, sputum production, and wheezing. Pulmonary function tests demonstrate airflow obstruction that is not fully reversible, distinguishing COPD from asthma, including CVA.

8. Interstitial Lung Disease (ILD):

ILD encompasses a heterogeneous group of diffuse parenchymal lung disorders, characterized by inflammation and fibrosis of the lung interstitium. While cough is a common symptom of ILD, it is often accompanied by dyspnea, exertional hypoxemia, and fine inspiratory crackles on auscultation. HRCT of the chest reveals characteristic patterns of lung fibrosis or inflammation, aiding in the diagnosis of specific ILD subtypes.

Conclusion:

In conclusion, the differential diagnosis of cough-variant asthma encompasses a wide array of respiratory and non-respiratory conditions, each with distinct clinical features, diagnostic criteria, and management strategies. By employing a systematic approach to evaluating patients with chronic cough, clinicians can effectively differentiate CVA from other potential causes and tailor treatment interventions accordingly. Collaboration between pulmonologists, allergists, gastroenterologists, and other specialists may be necessary to optimize patient care and outcomes in complex cases of chronic cough.

Importance of Early Detection and Diagnosis in Cough-Variant Asthma

Early detection and diagnosis play a pivotal role in the management and prognosis of cough-variant asthma (CVA), a unique clinical phenotype characterized by chronic cough as the predominant symptom. Timely recognition of CVA enables healthcare providers to initiate appropriate interventions, optimize treatment strategies, and mitigate the risk of disease progression and complications. The importance of early detection and diagnosis in CVA is underscored by several key factors:

1. Preventing Disease Progression: Early detection allows for timely intervention to prevent the progression of CVA to more severe forms of asthma or the development of irreversible airway remodeling. By initiating treatment at the onset of symptoms, healthcare providers can suppress airway inflammation, reduce bronchial hyperresponsiveness, and preserve lung function in affected individuals.

2. Improving Quality of Life: Chronic cough associated with CVA can significantly impair patients' quality of life, leading to physical discomfort, social embarrassment, and psychological distress. Early diagnosis enables healthcare providers to address symptoms promptly, alleviate cough-related morbidity, and improve patients' overall well-being.

3. Reducing Healthcare Utilization: Delayed diagnosis of CVA may result in frequent healthcare visits, unnecessary diagnostic tests, and inappropriate use of medications for presumed causes of chronic cough. Early recognition of CVA allows for targeted interventions, reducing the need for repetitive evaluations and minimizing healthcare costs associated with misdiagnosis and ineffective treatments.

4. Tailoring Treatment Strategies: Accurate diagnosis of CVA facilitates the selection of appropriate treatment strategies tailored to individual patients' needs and preferences. By identifying specific triggers, comorbid conditions, and underlying inflammatory mechanisms, healthcare providers can optimize pharmacological and non-pharmacological interventions to achieve better symptom control and disease management.

5. Minimizing Exacerbations and Complications: Untreated or undertreated CVA may lead to recurrent exacerbations, worsening of symptoms, and increased risk of complications such as respiratory infections or bronchial hyperreactivity. Early intervention can reduce the frequency and severity of exacerbations, prevent respiratory complications, and improve long-term outcomes for patients with CVA.

6. Enhancing Patient Education and Empowerment: Early diagnosis provides an opportunity for patient education and empowerment, enabling individuals to better understand their condition, recognize potential triggers, and participate actively in self-management strategies. By fostering patient engagement and adherence to treatment regimens, healthcare providers can promote optimal disease control and long-term adherence to therapeutic interventions.

7. Facilitating Monitoring and Follow-up: Early detection of CVA allows for timely initiation of monitoring and follow-up to assess treatment response, adjust therapy as needed, and identify emerging complications or comorbidities. Regular monitoring of symptoms, lung function, and medication adherence enables healthcare providers to optimize disease management and minimize the risk of disease exacerbations or relapses.

Conclusion: In conclusion, early detection and diagnosis are essential in the management of cough-variant asthma, enabling healthcare providers to initiate timely interventions, improve symptom control, and enhance patients' quality of life. By recognizing the importance of early intervention, healthcare providers can optimize treatment outcomes, reduce healthcare utilization, and minimize the burden of disease on affected individuals and healthcare systems. Emphasizing the importance of early detection and diagnosis in CVA underscores the significance of proactive screening, comprehensive evaluation, and patient-centered care in optimizing outcomes for patients with chronic cough.

CHAPTER 2: PATHOPHYSIOLOGY OF COUGH-VARIANT ASTHMA

Airway Inflammation and Remodeling in Cough-Variant Asthma

Cough-variant asthma (CVA) is characterized by chronic cough as the predominant symptom, which is driven by underlying airway inflammation and remodeling. Understanding the pathophysiological mechanisms of airway inflammation and remodeling in CVA is crucial for elucidating disease progression, identifying therapeutic targets, and optimizing management strategies. This section explores the intricate interplay between airway inflammation and remodeling in CVA, highlighting key cellular and molecular processes involved.

1. Airway Inflammation in Cough-Variant Asthma:

The hallmark feature of CVA is chronic inflammation of the airways, characterized by infiltration of inflammatory cells, release of pro-inflammatory mediators, and activation of immune pathways. Unlike classic asthma, where inflammation may be more diffuse and involve both large and small airways, CVA predominantly affects the small airways, contributing to the unique clinical phenotype of chronic cough.

1.1 Cellular Components of Airway Inflammation:

Several inflammatory cell types play a central role in driving airway inflammation in CVA, including eosinophils, mast cells, T lymphocytes, and neutrophils. Eosinophils are prominent in the airways of patients with CVA, releasing inflammatory cytokines and lipid mediators that promote airway hyperresponsiveness and mucus production. Mast cells contribute to bronchoconstriction and airway remodeling through the release of histamine, leukotrienes, and proteases. T lymphocytes, particularly the Th2 subset, secrete cytokines such as interleukin-4 (IL-4), IL-5, and IL-13, which promote eosinophilic inflammation and IgE-mediated responses. Neutrophils may also be present in the airways of patients with CVA, particularly during exacerbations or in severe cases, contributing to airway obstruction and tissue damage.

1.2 Mediators of Airway Inflammation:

Various inflammatory mediators orchestrate the inflammatory response in CVA, amplifying immune activation and perpetuating airway inflammation. These mediators include cytokines, chemokines, leukotrienes, prostaglandins, and reactive oxygen species. Interleukins such as IL-4, IL-5, and IL-13 promote eosinophilic inflammation, mucus hypersecretion, and airway remodeling. Chemokines such as eotaxins and RANTES (regulated upon activation, normal T cell expressed and secreted) recruit eosinophils and other inflammatory cells to the airways. Leukotrienes and prostaglandins induce bronchoconstriction, airway edema, and mucus production, exacerbating respiratory symptoms in patients with CVA. Reactive oxygen species generated by activated inflammatory cells contribute to oxidative stress and tissue damage, further perpetuating the inflammatory cascade.

2. Airway Remodeling in Cough-Variant Asthma:

In addition to inflammation, airway remodeling is a hallmark feature of asthma, including CVA, characterized by structural changes in the airway wall, subepithelial fibrosis, and smooth muscle hypertrophy. These structural alterations contribute to airflow limitation, bronchial hyperresponsiveness, and irreversible changes in lung function, highlighting the importance of targeting airway remodeling in the management of CVA.

2.1 Structural Changes in the Airway Wall:

Airway remodeling in CVA encompasses multiple structural alterations in the airway wall, including thickening of the basement membrane, increased deposition of extracellular matrix proteins (e.g., collagen, fibronectin), and hypertrophy of smooth muscle cells. These changes result in narrowing of the airway lumen, reduced airway caliber, and increased resistance to airflow, contributing to symptoms such as cough, dyspnea, and wheezing. Thickening of the basement membrane, in particular, is a hallmark feature of airway remodeling in asthma, reflecting chronic inflammation and repair processes within the airway epithelium.

2.2 Subepithelial Fibrosis and Matrix Remodeling:

Subepithelial fibrosis, characterized by excessive deposition of collagen and other extracellular matrix proteins beneath the airway epithelium, is a key component of airway remodeling in CVA. This fibrotic process disrupts normal airway architecture, impairs mucociliary clearance, and perpetuates airway inflammation. Matrix metalloproteinases (MMPs) and tissue inhibitors of metalloproteinases (TIMPs) play a critical role in regulating matrix remodeling and turnover in the airway wall, with dysregulation of MMP/TIMP balance contributing to aberrant tissue repair and fibrosis in asthma.

2.3 Smooth Muscle Hypertrophy and Hyperplasia:

Smooth muscle hypertrophy and hyperplasia are prominent features of airway remodeling in asthma, including CVA, leading to increased contractility and bronchial hyperresponsiveness. Pro-inflammatory cytokines such as IL-13 and transforming growth factor-beta (TGF-β) promote smooth muscle proliferation and hypertrophy, exacerbating airway narrowing and airflow limitation. Additionally, neurotrophic factors released during inflammation may sensitize airway smooth muscle cells, amplifying bronchoconstrictor responses and enhancing the severity of respiratory symptoms in patients with CVA.

Conclusion:

In conclusion, airway inflammation and remodeling play a central role in the pathogenesis of cough-variant asthma, driving chronic cough and respiratory symptoms in affected individuals. Understanding the cellular and molecular mechanisms underlying airway inflammation and remodeling is crucial for developing targeted therapeutic interventions aimed at modulating immune responses, suppressing inflammation, and preventing structural changes in the airway wall. By elucidating the complex interplay between inflammation and remodeling in CVA, researchers and clinicians can advance our understanding of disease pathophysiology and improve outcomes for patients with this distinct clinical phenotype of asthma.

Role of Immunoglobulin E (IgE) in Cough-Variant Asthma

Immunoglobulin E (IgE) plays a crucial role in the

pathogenesis of asthma, including cough-variant asthma (CVA). As a key mediator of allergic reactions, IgE contributes to airway inflammation, bronchial hyperresponsiveness, and respiratory symptoms in patients with CVA. Understanding the role of IgE in CVA is essential for elucidating disease mechanisms, identifying potential therapeutic targets, and optimizing management strategies. This section explores the multifaceted role of IgE in CVA, highlighting its involvement in airway inflammation, sensitization to allergens, and immune dysregulation.

1. IgE-Mediated Immune Responses:

IgE is a subclass of immunoglobulin produced by plasma cells in response to exposure to allergens, pathogens, or environmental stimuli. Upon sensitization, allergen-specific IgE antibodies bind to high-affinity IgE receptors (FcεRI) expressed on the surface of mast cells, basophils, and other immune cells, triggering a cascade of inflammatory reactions. Cross-linking of IgE receptors by allergens induces degranulation of mast cells and release of inflammatory mediators, such as histamine, leukotrienes, and cytokines, leading to bronchoconstriction, mucus production, and airway inflammation.

2. Sensitization to Allergens:

In CVA, as in other forms of asthma, sensitization to allergens plays a pivotal role in triggering and perpetuating airway inflammation. Patients with CVA often have a history of atopic conditions, such as allergic rhinitis, eczema, or food allergies, indicating a predisposition to allergic sensitization. Common allergens implicated in CVA include house dust mites, pollen, animal dander, mold spores, and certain foods. Sensitization to these allergens results in the production of allergen-specific IgE antibodies, which bind to mast cells and trigger allergic reactions upon re-exposure to the allergen.

3. Airway Inflammation and IgE:

The binding of allergen-specific IgE antibodies to mast cells and basophils initiates a cascade of inflammatory events, culminating in airway inflammation and bronchoconstriction. Histamine released from activated mast cells induces bronchial smooth muscle contraction, mucosal edema, and increased vascular permeability, leading to airflow limitation and respiratory symptoms. Additionally, leukotrienes, prostaglandins, and cytokines released during the allergic response amplify airway inflammation, recruit inflammatory cells, and promote tissue remodeling in the airway wall.

4. IgE-Targeted Therapies:

Given the central role of IgE in the pathogenesis of asthma, including CVA, targeting IgE-mediated immune responses has emerged as a promising therapeutic approach for managing allergic asthma. Omalizumab, a monoclonal antibody that binds to circulating IgE antibodies and prevents their interaction with FcεRI receptors, has been approved for the treatment of moderate to severe allergic asthma. By sequestering free IgE antibodies and reducing their availability for binding to mast cells and basophils, omalizumab inhibits allergen-induced mast cell activation and attenuates airway inflammation, bronchial hyperresponsiveness, and asthma exacerbations.

5. Potential Biomarker of Disease Severity:

Measurement of serum IgE levels may serve as a useful biomarker of disease severity and treatment response in patients with CVA. Elevated serum IgE levels are often observed in patients with allergic asthma, reflecting the degree of allergic sensitization and the intensity of allergic inflammation in the airways. Monitoring changes in serum IgE levels over time may provide insights into disease progression, response to therapy, and the need for adjunctive treatments such as omalizumab.

6. Future Directions:

Further research is needed to elucidate the precise role of IgE in the pathogenesis of CVA and to explore novel therapeutic targets for modulating IgE-mediated immune responses. Emerging approaches, such as allergen-specific immunotherapy and biologic agents targeting IgE receptors or downstream signaling pathways, hold promise for improving outcomes in patients with CVA and reducing the burden of allergic asthma on affected individuals and healthcare systems.

Conclusion:

In conclusion, IgE-mediated immune responses play a central role in the pathogenesis of cough-variant asthma, contributing to airway inflammation, sensitization to allergens, and respiratory symptoms in affected individuals. Targeting IgE-mediated pathways represents a promising therapeutic strategy for managing allergic asthma, including CVA, and may provide opportunities for personalized treatment approaches tailored to individual patients' immune profiles and disease phenotypes. By elucidating the role of IgE in CVA and exploring novel therapeutic interventions, researchers and clinicians can advance our understanding of disease mechanisms and improve outcomes for patients with this distinct clinical phenotype of asthma.

Mast Cell Activation and Mediator Release in Cough-Variant Asthma

Mast cells are pivotal players in the pathophysiology of cough-variant asthma (CVA), contributing to airway inflammation, bronchial hyperresponsiveness, and respiratory symptoms through their activation and release of inflammatory mediators.

Understanding the mechanisms underlying mast cell activation and mediator release in CVA is essential for elucidating disease pathogenesis, identifying therapeutic targets, and optimizing management strategies. This section explores the intricate interplay between mast cells and airway inflammation in CVA, highlighting key cellular and molecular processes involved in mast cell activation and mediator release.

1. Mast Cell Biology:

Mast cells are tissue-resident immune cells distributed throughout the body, particularly in mucosal and connective tissues, where they play a crucial role in allergic reactions, host defense, and tissue homeostasis. Mast cells are equipped with high-affinity IgE receptors (FcεRI) on their surface, allowing them to recognize and respond to allergens, pathogens, or other stimuli. Upon cross-linking of IgE receptors by allergens, mast cells undergo degranulation, releasing preformed mediators stored in intracellular granules and synthesizing de novo mediators in response to inflammatory signals.

2. Mechanisms of Mast Cell Activation:

Mast cell activation in CVA is triggered by allergen exposure, respiratory infections, environmental pollutants, or other inflammatory stimuli, leading to degranulation and release of inflammatory mediators. Allergen-specific IgE antibodies bound to FcεRI receptors on mast cells recognize and bind to allergens, initiating a signaling cascade that culminates in calcium influx, degranulation, and mediator release. In addition to IgE-mediated activation, mast cells can also be activated by non-IgE-dependent mechanisms, such as direct contact with pathogens, toll-like receptor (TLR) ligands, cytokines, or neuropeptides, further amplifying airway inflammation in CVA.

3. Preformed Mediators:

Mast cells store a plethora of preformed mediators within

their cytoplasmic granules, which are rapidly released upon degranulation to initiate an acute inflammatory response. These preformed mediators include histamine, proteases (e.g., tryptase, chymase), heparin, and cytokines (e.g., tumor necrosis factor-alpha [TNF-α]). Histamine is a potent vasodilator and bronchoconstrictor, promoting mucosal edema, smooth muscle contraction, and airflow limitation in the airways. Mast cell proteases contribute to tissue remodeling, mucus hypersecretion, and activation of other inflammatory cells, further perpetuating the inflammatory cascade in CVA.

4. Synthesized Mediators:

In addition to preformed mediators, mast cells also synthesize de novo mediators in response to inflammatory signals, amplifying the immune response and sustaining airway inflammation in CVA. These synthesized mediators include leukotrienes, prostaglandins, cytokines, chemokines, and growth factors, which are generated through the activation of intracellular signaling pathways, such as the arachidonic acid pathway, nuclear factor-kappa B (NF-κB) pathway, or mitogen-activated protein kinase (MAPK) pathway. Leukotrienes and prostaglandins induce bronchoconstriction, airway edema, and mucus production, while cytokines and chemokines recruit inflammatory cells and amplify the inflammatory response in the airways. Growth factors released by mast cells promote tissue repair, fibrosis, and airway remodeling, contributing to the chronicity of airway inflammation in CVA.

5. Regulation of Mast Cell Activation:

Mast cell activation and mediator release are tightly regulated by a balance of activating and inhibitory signals within the local microenvironment. Endogenous mediators, such as adenosine, prostaglandin E2 (PGE2), or corticosteroids, may modulate mast cell activation and limit excessive inflammation in the airways. Conversely, dysregulation of these regulatory mechanisms may contribute to aberrant mast cell activation and sustained airway inflammation in CVA. For example, downregulation of inhibitory receptors, such as the IgG FcγRIIB receptor, may enhance mast cell activation and exacerbate airway inflammation in asthma.

6. Therapeutic Implications:

Targeting mast cell activation and mediator release represents a promising therapeutic strategy for managing airway inflammation and respiratory symptoms in CVA. Pharmacological agents such as antihistamines, mast cell stabilizers, leukotriene receptor antagonists, and biologic agents targeting specific mast cell mediators (e.g., anti-IgE antibodies) have been investigated for their efficacy in attenuating mast cell activation and suppressing airway inflammation in asthma. Additionally, lifestyle modifications, such as allergen avoidance, environmental control measures, and dietary interventions, may help mitigate mast cell activation and reduce symptom exacerbations in patients with CVA.

Conclusion:

In conclusion, mast cell activation and mediator release play a central role in the pathogenesis of cough-variant asthma, contributing to airway inflammation, bronchial hyperresponsiveness, and respiratory symptoms in affected individuals. Understanding the mechanisms underlying mast cell activation and mediator release in CVA is essential for developing targeted therapeutic interventions aimed at modulating mast cell function, suppressing airway inflammation, and improving outcomes for patients with this distinct clinical phenotype of asthma. By elucidating the complex interplay between mast cells and airway inflammation in CVA, researchers and clinicians can advance our understanding of disease pathophysiology and develop personalized treatment approaches tailored to individual patients' immune profiles and disease severity.

Eosinophil Involvement in Cough-Variant Asthma

Eosinophils are key effector cells implicated in the pathogenesis of asthma, including cough-variant asthma (CVA). Their involvement in airway inflammation, tissue remodeling, and bronchial hyperresponsiveness underscores their significance in the pathophysiology of CVA. Understanding the role of eosinophils in CVA is vital for elucidating disease mechanisms, identifying therapeutic targets, and optimizing management strategies. This section explores the multifaceted involvement of eosinophils in CVA, highlighting their contributions to airway inflammation, cytokine release, and disease severity.

1. Eosinophil Recruitment and Activation:

Eosinophils are granulocytic leukocytes primarily involved in host defense against parasitic infections and allergic responses. In CVA, eosinophil recruitment to the airways is driven by various chemotactic factors, including eotaxins, interleukin-5 (IL-5), and leukotriene B4 (LTB4), released in response to allergen exposure or inflammatory stimuli. Once recruited, eosinophils become activated, releasing a myriad of pro-inflammatory mediators, cytokines, and cytotoxic proteins that contribute to airway inflammation and tissue damage.

2. Airway Inflammation and Eosinophilic Infiltration:

Eosinophilic inflammation is a hallmark feature of asthma, including CVA, characterized by the accumulation of eosinophils within the airway mucosa, submucosa, and lumen. In patients with CVA, eosinophilic infiltration of the airways correlates with disease severity, symptom frequency, and bronchial hyperresponsiveness. Eosinophils release cytotoxic granule proteins, such as eosinophil peroxidase (EPO) and major basic protein (MBP), which induce epithelial damage, mucus hypersecretion, and airway remodeling, perpetuating the inflammatory cascade in CVA.

3. Cytokine and Chemokine Production:

Eosinophils are potent producers of cytokines and chemokines that modulate immune responses and recruit other inflammatory cells to the airways. IL-5, a key cytokine involved in eosinophilopoiesis and survival, promotes eosinophil recruitment, activation, and survival in the airways of patients with CVA. Additionally, eosinophils release cytokines such as IL-4, IL-13, and tumor necrosis factor-alpha (TNF-α), which further amplify airway inflammation, promote IgE production, and induce mucus production by airway epithelial cells.

4. Role in Tissue Remodeling and Fibrosis:

Eosinophils contribute to airway remodeling and fibrosis through their release of profibrotic mediators and interaction with other inflammatory cells. Eosinophil-derived transforming growth factor-beta (TGF-β) stimulates fibroblast activation, collagen deposition, and extracellular matrix remodeling in the airway wall, leading to subepithelial fibrosis and increased airway smooth muscle mass. Furthermore, eosinophils release matrix metalloproteinases (MMPs) and tissue inhibitors of metalloproteinases (TIMPs), which regulate extracellular matrix turnover and tissue remodeling in the airways of patients with CVA.

5. Biomarker of Disease Severity:

Eosinophilic inflammation serves as a valuable biomarker of disease severity and treatment response in CVA. Peripheral blood eosinophil counts and sputum eosinophil percentages are frequently elevated in patients with CVA, reflecting the degree of airway inflammation and the intensity of allergic responses. Monitoring changes in eosinophilic inflammation over time may provide insights into disease progression, response to therapy, and the need for adjunctive treatments such as corticosteroids or biologic agents targeting eosinophilic pathways.

6. Therapeutic Implications:

Targeting eosinophilic inflammation represents a promising therapeutic strategy for managing airway inflammation and respiratory symptoms in CVA. Pharmacological agents such as corticosteroids, leukotriene receptor antagonists, and biologic agents targeting eosinophil-specific cytokines (e.g., anti-IL-5 antibodies) have been investigated for their efficacy in attenuating eosinophilic inflammation and suppressing airway hyperresponsiveness in asthma. Additionally, lifestyle modifications, such as allergen avoidance, smoking cessation, and environmental control measures, may help mitigate eosinophilic inflammation and reduce symptom exacerbations in patients with CVA.

Conclusion:

In conclusion, eosinophilic inflammation plays a central role in the pathogenesis of cough-variant asthma, contributing to airway inflammation, tissue remodeling, and bronchial hyperresponsiveness in affected individuals. Understanding the multifaceted involvement of eosinophils in CVA is essential for developing targeted therapeutic interventions aimed at modulating eosinophilic pathways, suppressing airway inflammation, and improving outcomes for patients with this distinct clinical phenotype of asthma. By elucidating the complex interplay between eosinophils and airway inflammation in CVA, researchers and clinicians can advance our understanding of disease pathophysiology and develop personalized treatment approaches tailored to individual patients' immune profiles and disease severity.

Role of T-helper Cells (Th2) in Cough-Variant Asthma

T-helper cells, particularly the Th2 subset, play a pivotal role in orchestrating the immune response in asthma, including cough-variant asthma (CVA). Th2 cells drive airway inflammation, eosinophilic infiltration, and production of pro-inflammatory cytokines, contributing to respiratory symptoms and airway hyperresponsiveness in patients with CVA. Understanding the role of Th2 cells in CVA is essential for elucidating disease mechanisms, identifying therapeutic targets, and optimizing management strategies. This section explores the multifaceted involvement of Th2 cells in CVA, highlighting their contributions to airway inflammation, cytokine release, and disease pathogenesis.

1. Th2 Cell Differentiation and Activation:

Th2 cells arise from naive CD4+ T lymphocytes upon activation by antigen-presenting cells (APCs) in the context of allergens, microbial pathogens, or other inflammatory stimuli. Th2 cell differentiation is driven by cytokines such as interleukin-4 (IL-4), which promote the expression of lineage-specific transcription factors (e.g., GATA3) and induce a Th2 phenotype characterized by the production of IL-4, IL-5, and IL-13. Once activated, Th2 cells migrate to the airways and release cytokines that modulate immune responses, recruit inflammatory cells, and promote airway inflammation in CVA.

2. Airway Inflammation and Th2 Cytokines:

Th2 cytokines, particularly IL-4, IL-5, and IL-13, play a central role in driving airway inflammation and eosinophilic infiltration in CVA. IL-4 promotes B cell class switching to IgE, enhancing allergic sensitization and IgE-mediated responses in the airways. IL-5 stimulates eosinophilopoiesis, recruitment, and survival, amplifying eosinophilic inflammation and tissue damage in the airways of patients with CVA. IL-13 induces mucus hypersecretion, goblet cell metaplasia, and airway remodeling, contributing to respiratory symptoms and airflow limitation in CVA.

3. Regulation of IgE-Mediated Responses:

Th2 cells regulate IgE-mediated immune responses through their production of IL-4, which promotes IgE class switching in B cells and enhances IgE production by plasma cells. Elevated serum IgE levels are frequently observed in patients with CVA, reflecting the degree of Th2-driven allergic inflammation in the airways. IgE antibodies bound to mast cells and basophils initiate allergic reactions upon allergen exposure, inducing mast cell degranulation, release of inflammatory mediators, and bronchial hyperresponsiveness in patients with CVA.

4. Interaction with Other Immune Cells:

Th2 cells interact with other immune cells, including eosinophils, mast cells, dendritic cells, and epithelial cells, to orchestrate the inflammatory response in CVA. Eosinophils and mast cells respond to Th2 cytokines by releasing pro-inflammatory mediators and amplifying airway inflammation in the lungs. Dendritic cells present antigens to Th2 cells, initiating adaptive immune responses and promoting allergic sensitization in the airways. Epithelial cells produce cytokines and chemokines in response to Th2-derived signals, further perpetuating airway inflammation and remodeling in CVA.

5. Therapeutic Implications:

Targeting Th2-driven immune responses represents a promising therapeutic strategy for managing airway inflammation and respiratory symptoms in CVA. Pharmacological agents such as corticosteroids, leukotriene receptor antagonists, and biologic agents targeting Th2 cytokines (e.g., anti-IL-4, anti-IL-5, anti-IL-13 antibodies) have been investigated for their efficacy in attenuating Th2-driven inflammation and suppressing airway hyperresponsiveness in asthma. Additionally, lifestyle modifications, such as allergen avoidance, environmental control measures, and dietary interventions, may help mitigate Th2-mediated inflammation and reduce symptom exacerbations in patients with CVA.

Conclusion:

In conclusion, Th2 cells play a central role in the pathogenesis of cough-variant asthma, contributing to airway inflammation, eosinophilic infiltration, and respiratory symptoms in affected individuals. Understanding the multifaceted involvement of Th2 cells in CVA is essential for developing targeted therapeutic interventions aimed at modulating Th2-driven immune responses, suppressing airway inflammation, and improving outcomes for patients with this distinct clinical phenotype of asthma. By elucidating the complex interplay between Th2 cells and airway inflammation in CVA, researchers and clinicians can advance our understanding of disease pathophysiology and develop personalized treatment approaches tailored to individual patients' immune profiles and disease severity.

Neurogenic Inflammation and the Cough Reflex in Cough-Variant Asthma

Neurogenic inflammation and the cough reflex play crucial roles in the pathogenesis of cough-variant asthma (CVA), contributing to the initiation and perpetuation of chronic cough as the predominant symptom. Understanding the mechanisms underlying neurogenic inflammation and the cough reflex in CVA is essential for elucidating disease mechanisms, identifying therapeutic targets, and optimizing management strategies. This section explores the multifaceted involvement of neurogenic inflammation and the cough reflex in CVA, highlighting their contributions to airway hypersensitivity, neuronal activation, and respiratory symptoms.

1. Neurogenic Inflammation:

Neurogenic inflammation refers to the inflammatory response initiated by the activation of sensory nerves, particularly C-fiber nociceptors, in the airways. In CVA, neurogenic inflammation is triggered by various stimuli, including allergens, irritants, respiratory infections, and inflammatory mediators, leading to the release of neuropeptides such as substance P, neurokinins, and calcitonin gene-related peptide (CGRP) from sensory nerve terminals. These neuropeptides induce vasodilation, plasma extravasation, and recruitment of inflammatory cells, amplifying airway inflammation and exacerbating respiratory symptoms in patients with CVA.

2. Role of Sensory Nerves:

Sensory nerves, particularly vagal C-fiber nociceptors, play a pivotal role in detecting and transmitting noxious stimuli from the airways to the central nervous system. In CVA, activation of sensory nerves by allergens, airway inflammation, or mechanical stimuli triggers the release of neurotransmitters such as substance P and neurokinins, which modulate neuronal excitability and initiate the cough reflex. Additionally, neurotrophic factors released during inflammation may sensitize sensory nerves, amplifying their responsiveness to stimuli and exacerbating cough hypersensitivity in patients with CVA.

3. Cough Reflex Pathway:

The cough reflex is a protective mechanism that helps clear the airways of irritants, secretions, and foreign particles. In

CVA, the cough reflex is hypersensitive and exaggerated, leading to persistent, non-productive cough as the primary symptom. The cough reflex pathway involves sensory receptors in the airway epithelium, afferent nerve fibers (vagal C-fibers), central processing centers in the brainstem (cough center), and efferent nerve fibers innervating respiratory muscles and airway smooth muscle. Activation of sensory nerves by noxious stimuli triggers a reflexive cough response mediated by rapid expiration, glottal closure, and contraction of expiratory muscles, leading to coughing paroxysms in patients with CVA.

4. Neurotransmitters and Neuropeptides:

Neurotransmitters and neuropeptides released from sensory nerves modulate neuronal excitability and cough responsiveness in CVA. Substance P, neurokinins, and CGRP released from sensory nerve terminals sensitize cough receptors and enhance cough reflex sensitivity in response to allergens, irritants, or inflammatory mediators. Additionally, glutamate and gamma-aminobutyric acid (GABA) released within the cough reflex pathway modulate neuronal activity and cough responsiveness, influencing the intensity and frequency of coughing episodes in patients with CVA.

5. Therapeutic Implications:

Targeting neurogenic inflammation and the cough reflex represents a promising therapeutic strategy for managing chronic cough and respiratory symptoms in CVA. Pharmacological agents such as neurokinin receptor antagonists, transient receptor potential (TRP) channel antagonists, and cough suppressants (e.g., opioids, gabapentinoids) have been investigated for their efficacy in attenuating cough hypersensitivity and suppressing coughing paroxysms in patients with CVA. Additionally, non-pharmacological interventions, such as breathing exercises, speech therapy, and cognitive-behavioral therapy, may help modulate cough reflex sensitivity and improve cough-related quality of life in patients with CVA.

Conclusion:

In conclusion, neurogenic inflammation and the cough reflex play crucial roles in the pathogenesis of cough-variant asthma, contributing to airway hypersensitivity, neuronal activation, and respiratory symptoms in affected individuals. Understanding the multifaceted involvement of neurogenic inflammation and the cough reflex in CVA is essential for developing targeted therapeutic interventions aimed at modulating sensory nerve function, suppressing cough reflex sensitivity, and improving outcomes for patients with this distinct clinical phenotype of asthma. By elucidating the complex interplay between neurogenic inflammation, sensory nerves, and the cough reflex in CVA, researchers and clinicians can advance our understanding of disease pathophysiology and develop personalized treatment approaches tailored to individual patients' cough profiles and disease severity.

Airway Hyperresponsiveness in Cough-Variant Asthma

Airway hyperresponsiveness (AHR) is a hallmark feature of asthma, including cough-variant asthma (CVA), characterized by exaggerated bronchoconstrictor responses to various stimuli. AHR contributes to respiratory symptoms, airflow limitation, and cough hypersensitivity in patients with CVA. Understanding the mechanisms underlying AHR in CVA is essential for elucidating disease pathogenesis, identifying therapeutic targets, and optimizing management strategies. This section explores the multifaceted involvement of AHR in CVA, highlighting its contributions to bronchial smooth muscle contraction, airway remodeling, and respiratory symptoms.

1. Bronchial Smooth Muscle Contraction:

AHR in CVA is primarily driven by excessive contraction of bronchial smooth muscle cells in response to various stimuli, such as allergens, irritants, cold air, exercise, or respiratory infections. Bronchial smooth muscle hyperreactivity results from dysregulation of calcium signaling, altered expression of contractile proteins, and enhanced responsiveness to contractile agonists, leading to increased airway narrowing and airflow limitation. In patients with CVA, bronchial smooth muscle contraction contributes to respiratory symptoms, cough hypersensitivity, and airflow obstruction, exacerbating disease severity and impairing lung function.

2. Inflammatory Mediators and Cytokines:

Inflammatory mediators and cytokines released during airway inflammation play a central role in modulating airway smooth muscle function and promoting AHR in CVA. Pro-inflammatory cytokines such as interleukin-13 (IL-13) and tumor necrosis factor-alpha (TNF-α) induce bronchial smooth muscle contraction, airway remodeling, and mucus hypersecretion, exacerbating respiratory symptoms and coughing paroxysms in patients with CVA. Additionally, leukotrienes, prostaglandins, and histamine released during allergic reactions enhance bronchial smooth muscle reactivity and contribute to AHR in CVA.

3. Airway Remodeling and Structural Changes:

Airway remodeling, characterized by structural alterations in the airway wall, subepithelial fibrosis, and smooth muscle hypertrophy, contributes to AHR in CVA. Thickening of the basement membrane, increased deposition of extracellular matrix proteins (e.g., collagen, fibronectin), and hypertrophy of bronchial smooth muscle cells reduce airway caliber and increase airway resistance, enhancing bronchoconstrictor responses to various stimuli. Additionally, subepithelial fibrosis disrupts normal airway architecture, impairs mucociliary clearance, and exacerbates airflow limitation in patients with CVA, further amplifying AHR and respiratory symptoms.

4. Neural Mechanisms:

Neural mechanisms, including autonomic nervous system dysfunction, vagal hyperreactivity, and sensory nerve activation, contribute to AHR in CVA. Parasympathetic activation induces bronchoconstriction and airway hyperreactivity through the release of acetylcholine and activation of muscarinic receptors on bronchial smooth muscle cells. Additionally, sensory nerve activation by allergens, irritants, or inflammatory mediators triggers the release of neuropeptides such as substance P and neurokinins, which modulate bronchomotor tone and enhance AHR in patients with CVA.

5. Therapeutic Implications:

Targeting AHR represents a cornerstone of asthma management, including CVA, aimed at reducing respiratory symptoms, improving lung function, and enhancing quality of life in affected individuals. Pharmacological agents such as bronchodilators (e.g., β2-adrenergic agonists, anticholinergics), corticosteroids, leukotriene receptor antagonists, and biologic agents targeting inflammatory pathways (e.g., anti-IL-5 antibodies) have been investigated for their efficacy in attenuating AHR and suppressing airway inflammation in CVA. Additionally, non-pharmacological interventions, such as allergen avoidance, smoking cessation, and respiratory rehabilitation, may help mitigate AHR and improve lung function in patients with CVA.

Conclusion:

In conclusion, airway hyperresponsiveness is a key feature of cough-variant asthma, contributing to respiratory symptoms, cough hypersensitivity, and airflow limitation in affected individuals. Understanding the multifaceted involvement of AHR in CVA is essential for developing targeted therapeutic interventions aimed at modulating bronchial smooth muscle function, suppressing airway inflammation, and improving outcomes for patients with this distinct clinical phenotype of asthma. By elucidating the complex interplay between inflammatory mediators, neural mechanisms, and airway remodeling in CVA, researchers and clinicians can advance our understanding of disease pathophysiology and develop personalized treatment approaches tailored to individual patients' AHR profiles and disease severity.

Genetic Predisposition in Cough-Variant Asthma

Genetic predisposition plays a significant role in the pathogenesis and clinical manifestation of cough-variant asthma (CVA), influencing susceptibility to environmental triggers, airway inflammation, and bronchial hyperresponsiveness. Understanding the genetic determinants of CVA is essential for elucidating disease mechanisms, identifying biomarkers, and developing personalized treatment strategies. This section explores the complex interplay between genetic factors and CVA, highlighting key genetic variants, susceptibility genes, and gene-environment interactions implicated in disease pathogenesis.

1. Genetic Variants Associated with CVA:

Genome-wide association studies (GWAS) and candidate gene studies have identified several genetic variants associated with CVA susceptibility, disease severity, and treatment response. Single nucleotide polymorphisms (SNPs) in genes encoding inflammatory cytokines (e.g., interleukin-4 [IL-4], interleukin-13 [IL-13], tumor necrosis factor-alpha [TNF-α]), airway smooth muscle proteins (e.g., beta-2 adrenergic receptor [β2-AR]), and epithelial barrier proteins (e.g., claudins, desmosomes) have been implicated in the pathogenesis of CVA. Additionally, genetic variants in genes involved in mucin production, oxidative stress, and airway remodeling pathways may modulate disease susceptibility and severity in patients with CVA.

2. Susceptibility Genes and Pathways:

Susceptibility genes and biological pathways involved in airway inflammation, immune regulation, and bronchial hyperresponsiveness contribute to the genetic predisposition to CVA. Th2-associated cytokine genes (e.g., IL-4, IL-13) play a central role in promoting allergic sensitization, eosinophilic inflammation, and mucus hypersecretion in the airways of patients with CVA. Genetic variants in genes encoding components of the innate immune system (e.g., toll-like receptors [TLRs], pattern recognition receptors [PRRs]) may influence susceptibility to respiratory infections and exacerbations in CVA. Furthermore, genes involved in bronchial smooth muscle contraction (e.g., β2-AR, muscarinic receptors) and airway remodeling (e.g., matrix metalloproteinases [MMPs], tissue inhibitors of metalloproteinases [TIMPs]) modulate bronchial hyperresponsiveness and disease progression in CVA.

3. Gene-Environment Interactions:

Gene-environment interactions play a critical role in shaping the clinical phenotype and natural history of CVA, whereby genetic susceptibility factors interact with environmental triggers to influence disease onset, progression, and treatment response. Environmental exposures such as allergens, pollutants, respiratory infections, and occupational irritants may interact with genetic variants in inflammatory cytokine genes (e.g., IL-4, IL-13), airway epithelial genes (e.g., claudins, mucins), and bronchial smooth muscle genes (e.g., β2-AR) to exacerbate airway inflammation, bronchial hyperresponsiveness, and respiratory symptoms in patients with CVA. Additionally, lifestyle factors such as smoking, diet, physical activity, and psychosocial stress may modulate gene expression, epigenetic modifications, and immune responses in CVA, further influencing disease susceptibility and severity.

4. Familial Aggregation and Heritability:

Familial aggregation studies have demonstrated a genetic component to the inheritance of asthma, including CVA, with a higher prevalence of asthma and allergic conditions observed among first-degree relatives of affected individuals. Twin and family-based studies have estimated the heritability of asthma to be approximately 30-70%, indicating a significant genetic contribution to disease susceptibility and phenotype variability. Genome-wide linkage and association studies have identified chromosomal regions and candidate genes associated with asthma susceptibility loci, providing insights into the genetic architecture of CVA and potential targets for future research and therapeutic intervention.

5. Clinical Implications and Future Directions:

Understanding the genetic predisposition to CVA has important clinical implications for risk stratification, disease management, and precision medicine approaches. Genetic profiling and biomarker testing may help identify patients at increased risk of CVA, guide treatment decisions, and predict treatment response to bronchodilators, corticosteroids, and biologic agents targeting specific inflammatory pathways. Additionally, genetic counseling and family history assessment may help elucidate the inheritance pattern of asthma and allergic conditions, inform patient education, and facilitate early intervention strategies to mitigate environmental exposures and prevent disease exacerbations in high-risk individuals. Further research is needed to elucidate the genetic determinants of CVA, validate genetic biomarkers, and translate genetic discoveries into clinical practice to improve outcomes and quality of life for patients with this distinct clinical phenotype of asthma.

Conclusion:

In conclusion, genetic predisposition plays a significant role in the pathogenesis and clinical manifestation of cough-variant asthma, influencing susceptibility to environmental triggers, airway inflammation, and bronchial hyperresponsiveness in affected individuals. Understanding the complex interplay between genetic factors, environmental exposures, and disease phenotype variability is essential for elucidating disease mechanisms, identifying biomarkers, and developing personalized treatment strategies tailored to individual patients' genetic profiles and disease severity. By advancing our understanding of the genetic determinants of CVA, researchers and clinicians can pave the way for precision medicine approaches aimed at optimizing disease management and improving outcomes for patients with this distinct clinical phenotype of asthma.

CHAPTER 3: TRIGGER FACTORS AND ENVIRONMENTAL INFLUENCES

Allergens and Allergic Sensitization in Cough-Variant Asthma

Cough-variant asthma (CVA) is characterized by chronic cough as the predominant symptom, often triggered by exposure to allergens and associated with underlying airway inflammation and bronchial hyperresponsiveness. Allergens play a pivotal role in the pathogenesis of CVA, driving allergic sensitization, airway inflammation, and respiratory symptoms in susceptible individuals. Understanding the diverse array of allergens implicated in CVA and the mechanisms underlying allergic sensitization is essential for elucidating disease mechanisms, identifying triggers, and optimizing management strategies. This section explores the multifaceted relationship between allergens, allergic sensitization, and CVA, highlighting key allergenic triggers, immune responses, and therapeutic implications.

1. Common Allergenic Triggers:

A wide range of allergens can trigger coughing episodes and exacerbate respiratory symptoms in patients with CVA. Common allergenic triggers include:

- **Pollen:** Pollen grains from trees, grasses, and weeds are potent allergens that can induce allergic rhinitis and exacerbate respiratory symptoms in patients with CVA, particularly during pollen seasons.
- **Dust Mites:** Dust mites are microscopic arthropods commonly found in indoor environments, such as bedding, upholstered furniture, and carpeting, and can trigger allergic reactions in sensitized individuals with CVA.
- **Animal Dander:** Allergens from pets, such as cats, dogs, and rodents, can provoke allergic sensitization and exacerbate respiratory symptoms in patients with CVA exposed to animal dander.
- **Mold Spores:** Mold spores present in damp indoor environments, such as bathrooms, kitchens, and basements, can elicit allergic reactions and worsen respiratory symptoms in patients with CVA sensitive to mold allergens.
- **Cockroach Allergens:** Cockroach infestations in homes and urban environments can release allergenic proteins into the air, triggering allergic sensitization and exacerbating respiratory symptoms in susceptible individuals with CVA.

2. Mechanisms of Allergic Sensitization:

Allergic sensitization refers to the development of an immune response to allergens, characterized by the production of allergen-specific immunoglobulin E (IgE) antibodies and activation of Th2-mediated inflammatory pathways. The process of allergic sensitization involves several steps:

- **Allergen Exposure:** Initial exposure to allergens triggers immune responses in susceptible individuals, leading to allergen uptake by antigen-presenting cells (APCs) and activation of adaptive immune responses.
- **Antigen Presentation:** APCs, such as dendritic cells, present allergen-derived peptides to naive T cells in the context of major histocompatibility complex (MHC) class II molecules, initiating T cell activation and differentiation into allergen-specific Th2 cells.
- **Th2 Cell Activation:** Allergen-specific Th2 cells produce cytokines such as interleukin-4 (IL-4), interleukin-5 (IL-5), and interleukin-13 (IL-13), which promote B cell class switching to IgE, eosinophilic inflammation, and mucus hypersecretion in the airways.
- **B Cell Activation:** Allergen-specific Th2 cells provide help to B cells, promoting their differentiation into IgE-producing plasma cells and secretion of allergen-specific IgE antibodies.
- **IgE-Mediated Responses:** Allergen-specific IgE antibodies bind to high-affinity IgE receptors (FcεRI) on mast cells and basophils, sensitizing these cells to subsequent allergen exposures and triggering immediate hypersensitivity reactions upon allergen re-exposure.

3. Role of Allergen-Induced Inflammation:

Allergen-induced inflammation plays a central role in the pathogenesis of CVA, contributing to airway inflammation, bronchial hyperresponsiveness, and cough hypersensitivity. Allergens trigger the release of pro-inflammatory cytokines, chemokines, and inflammatory mediators, which recruit inflammatory cells (e.g., eosinophils, mast cells, T cells) to the airways and promote allergic inflammation. The activation of mast cells and eosinophils by allergen-specific IgE antibodies leads to the release of inflammatory mediators such as histamine, leukotrienes, and cytokines, which induce bronchoconstriction, airway edema, and mucus production, exacerbating coughing episodes and respiratory symptoms in patients with CVA.

4. Diagnostic Implications:

Identification of allergenic triggers and assessment of allergic sensitization are important components of the diagnostic evaluation and management of CVA. Allergy testing, including skin prick tests and serum-specific IgE assays, can help identify allergens responsible for triggering coughing episodes and exacerbating respiratory symptoms in patients with CVA. Additionally, monitoring changes in allergen-specific IgE levels and eosinophil counts over time may provide insights into disease progression, treatment response, and the need for allergen avoidance strategies or immunomodulatory therapies in patients with CVA.

5. Therapeutic Strategies:

Management of CVA involves both allergen avoidance strategies and pharmacological interventions aimed at reducing airway inflammation, bronchial hyperresponsiveness, and respiratory symptoms. Allergen avoidance measures, such as minimizing exposure to indoor allergens (e.g., dust mites, animal dander, mold), implementing environmental control measures (e.g., air filtration, mattress and pillow encasements), and adopting lifestyle modifications (e.g., pet restrictions, humidity control), may help mitigate allergen-induced inflammation and reduce coughing episodes in patients with CVA. Pharmacological interventions, including inhaled corticosteroids, bronchodilators (e.g., β2-agonists), leukotriene receptor antagonists, and biologic agents targeting Th2-mediated pathways (e.g., anti-IgE antibodies, anti-IL-5 antibodies), can help suppress airway inflammation, alleviate respiratory symptoms, and improve quality of life in patients with CVA sensitized to allergens.

Conclusion:

In conclusion, allergens play a central role in the pathogenesis of cough-variant asthma, driving allergic sensitization, airway inflammation, and respiratory symptoms in susceptible individuals. Understanding the mechanisms underlying allergic sensitization and allergen-induced inflammation is essential for elucidating disease mechanisms, identifying triggers, and optimizing management strategies for patients with CVA. By targeting allergenic triggers, modulating immune responses, and adopting personalized treatment approaches tailored to individual patients' allergic sensitivities and disease severity, clinicians can improve outcomes and quality of life for patients with this distinct clinical phenotype of asthma.

Respiratory Infections and their Impact on Cough-Variant Asthma

Respiratory infections represent a significant trigger and exacerbating factor for cough-variant asthma (CVA), contributing to airway inflammation, bronchial hyperresponsiveness, and respiratory symptoms in affected individuals. Understanding the complex interplay between respiratory infections and CVA is essential for elucidating disease mechanisms, identifying exacerbating factors, and optimizing management strategies. This section explores the multifaceted relationship between respiratory infections, immune responses, and CVA, highlighting key viral and bacterial pathogens, host immune responses, and therapeutic implications.

1. Viral Respiratory Infections:

Viral respiratory infections, particularly those caused by

rhinoviruses, respiratory syncytial virus (RSV), influenza viruses, and coronaviruses, are common triggers of acute exacerbations and worsening of respiratory symptoms in patients with CVA. Rhinoviruses, in particular, are implicated in the majority of viral-induced asthma exacerbations, affecting both children and adults with CVA. Viral respiratory infections can exacerbate airway inflammation, trigger bronchospasm, and impair lung function in patients with CVA, leading to coughing episodes, wheezing, and dyspnea.

2. Mechanisms of Viral-Induced Exacerbations:

Viral respiratory infections induce airway inflammation and immune responses through multiple mechanisms, including:

- **Direct Viral Effects:** Viruses infect airway epithelial cells, triggering innate immune responses, interferon production, and recruitment of inflammatory cells to the airways.
- **Indirect Effects:** Viral-induced epithelial damage, release of pro-inflammatory cytokines, and activation of Th2-mediated inflammatory pathways contribute to airway inflammation, bronchial hyperresponsiveness, and respiratory symptoms in patients with CVA.
- **Immune Responses:** Host immune responses to viral infections involve activation of dendritic cells, macrophages, and lymphocytes, leading to the release of cytokines, chemokines, and inflammatory mediators that promote airway inflammation and exacerbate asthma symptoms.

3. Bacterial Respiratory Infections:

Bacterial respiratory infections, such as those caused by Streptococcus pneumoniae, Haemophilus influenzae, and Moraxella catarrhalis, can also exacerbate airway inflammation and respiratory symptoms in patients with CVA, particularly in individuals with underlying airway hyperresponsiveness and impaired mucociliary clearance. Bacterial respiratory infections may complicate viral-induced exacerbations of CVA, leading to secondary bacterial pneumonia, sinusitis, or exacerbation of chronic bronchitis.

4. Host Immune Responses:

Host immune responses to respiratory infections play a critical role in the pathogenesis and clinical manifestation of CVA. Innate immune responses, including activation of toll-like receptors (TLRs), pattern recognition receptors (PRRs), and production of antiviral cytokines (e.g., interferons), provide initial defense against viral and bacterial pathogens, limiting viral replication and spread within the airways. Adaptive immune responses, mediated by T lymphocytes, B lymphocytes, and antigen-presenting cells, help clear viral and bacterial pathogens, promote resolution of inflammation, and prevent recurrent infections in patients with CVA.

5. Impact on Disease Severity:

Respiratory infections can significantly impact the severity and natural history of CVA, leading to acute exacerbations, worsening of respiratory symptoms, and impaired lung function in affected individuals. Viral-induced exacerbations of CVA are associated with increased healthcare utilization, medication use, and risk of hospitalization, highlighting the clinical significance of respiratory infections as exacerbating factors in patients with CVA. Bacterial superinfections, secondary to viral respiratory infections or underlying airway inflammation, may further complicate the clinical course of CVA, necessitating prompt diagnosis and appropriate antimicrobial therapy to prevent disease progression and complications.

6. Therapeutic Implications:

Management of respiratory infections in patients with CVA involves a combination of supportive care, pharmacological interventions, and preventive measures aimed at reducing symptom severity, preventing complications, and improving outcomes. Treatment strategies may include:

- **Antiviral Therapy:** Antiviral medications, such as neuraminidase inhibitors (e.g., oseltamivir, zanamivir), may be indicated for the treatment of influenza virus infections in patients with CVA, particularly those at high risk of complications.
- **Antibiotic Therapy:** Antibiotics may be prescribed for bacterial respiratory infections, such as acute exacerbations of chronic bronchitis or bacterial pneumonia, in patients with CVA, based on clinical presentation, severity of symptoms, and microbiological testing.
- **Bronchodilators:** Short-acting bronchodilators (e.g., β2-agonists) may provide symptomatic relief of coughing, wheezing, and dyspnea associated with viral-induced exacerbations of CVA, improving airflow and lung function.
- **Corticosteroids:** Systemic corticosteroids may be used to reduce airway inflammation, bronchial hyperresponsiveness, and exacerbation severity in patients with CVA experiencing viral-induced exacerbations or worsening of respiratory symptoms.

Conclusion:

In conclusion, respiratory infections represent significant triggers and exacerbating factors for cough-variant asthma, contributing to airway inflammation, bronchial hyperresponsiveness, and respiratory symptoms in affected individuals. Understanding the complex interplay between viral and bacterial pathogens, host immune responses, and disease severity is essential for elucidating disease mechanisms, identifying exacerbating factors, and optimizing management strategies for patients with CVA. By targeting respiratory infections, modulating immune responses, and adopting preventive measures, clinicians can reduce symptom severity, prevent complications, and improve outcomes for patients with this distinct clinical phenotype of asthma.

Environmental Pollutants and Their Impact on Cough-Variant Asthma

Environmental pollutants are significant contributors to respiratory diseases, including cough-variant asthma (CVA). Exposure to pollutants such as airborne particulate matter, nitrogen dioxide, ozone, volatile organic compounds, and tobacco smoke can exacerbate airway inflammation, bronchial hyperresponsiveness, and respiratory symptoms in individuals with CVA. Understanding the diverse array of environmental pollutants, their mechanisms of action, and their impact on CVA is crucial for elucidating disease mechanisms, identifying exacerbating factors, and optimizing management strategies. This section explores the multifaceted relationship between environmental pollutants and CVA, highlighting key pollutants, immune responses, and therapeutic implications.

1. Common Environmental Pollutants:

Several environmental pollutants are known to exacerbate respiratory symptoms and contribute to the development and progression of CVA. Common pollutants include:

- **Particulate Matter (PM):** Fine particulate matter (PM2.5) and coarse particulate matter (PM10) are airborne particles with diameters of 2.5 micrometers or smaller and 10 micrometers or smaller, respectively.

PM originates from various sources, including vehicle emissions, industrial activities, construction sites, and biomass burning, and can penetrate deep into the respiratory tract, triggering airway inflammation and exacerbating respiratory symptoms in individuals with CVA.

- **Nitrogen Dioxide (NO2):** Nitrogen dioxide is a gaseous air pollutant primarily emitted from motor vehicles, industrial processes, and combustion of fossil fuels. NO2 exposure can irritate the airways, induce oxidative stress, and exacerbate bronchial hyperresponsiveness in individuals with CVA, leading to coughing, wheezing, and dyspnea.
- **Ozone (O3):** Ozone is a reactive gas formed by the photochemical reaction of nitrogen oxides (NOx) and volatile organic compounds (VOCs) in the presence of sunlight. Ozone exposure can cause airway inflammation, epithelial injury, and bronchial hyperresponsiveness in individuals with CVA, exacerbating respiratory symptoms and impairing lung function.
- **Volatile Organic Compounds (VOCs):** VOCs are organic chemicals emitted from various sources, including motor vehicles, industrial processes, household products, and tobacco smoke. VOC exposure can trigger airway irritation, allergic sensitization, and exacerbation of respiratory symptoms in individuals with CVA sensitive to chemical irritants.
- **Tobacco Smoke:** Tobacco smoke is a complex mixture of toxic chemicals, including nicotine, carbon monoxide, tar, and carcinogens, which can cause airway inflammation, mucus hypersecretion, and bronchial hyperresponsiveness in individuals with CVA exposed to secondhand smoke or active smoking.

2. Mechanisms of Action:

Environmental pollutants exert their effects on the respiratory system through multiple mechanisms, including:

- **Airway Inflammation:** Pollutants such as PM, NO2, and ozone can induce airway inflammation by activating inflammatory cells (e.g., neutrophils, eosinophils), releasing pro-inflammatory cytokines (e.g., interleukin-6 [IL-6], interleukin-8 [IL-8]), and promoting oxidative stress-mediated damage to airway epithelial cells.
- **Bronchial Hyperresponsiveness:** Pollutants can enhance bronchial hyperresponsiveness by stimulating bronchial smooth muscle contraction, increasing airway resistance, and impairing lung function in individuals with CVA.
- **Oxidative Stress:** Pollutants such as ozone and VOCs can induce oxidative stress in the airways by generating reactive oxygen species (ROS), depleting antioxidant defenses, and promoting lipid peroxidation, leading to airway inflammation and tissue damage.
- **Immune Dysregulation:** Pollutants can disrupt immune responses by modulating cytokine production, impairing antigen presentation, and promoting Th2-mediated allergic inflammation in individuals with CVA.

3. Impact on Disease Severity:

Environmental pollutants can significantly impact the severity and natural history of CVA, leading to exacerbations, worsening of respiratory symptoms, and impaired lung function in affected individuals. Long-term exposure to high levels of pollutants, such as PM, NO2, and tobacco smoke, is associated with increased risk of asthma development, progression, and poor treatment outcomes in individuals with CVA. Pollutant-induced exacerbations of CVA are characterized by increased coughing episodes, wheezing, dyspnea, and reduced quality of life, necessitating prompt identification and mitigation of environmental exposures to improve disease control and outcomes.

4. Vulnerable Populations:

Certain populations may be particularly susceptible to the adverse effects of environmental pollutants on CVA, including:

- **Children:** Children with developing respiratory systems are more vulnerable to the effects of environmental pollutants, such as secondhand smoke exposure, indoor air pollution, and traffic-related air pollution, which can impair lung growth and development, increase asthma incidence, and exacerbate respiratory symptoms in children with CVA.
- **Elderly Individuals:** Elderly individuals with pre-existing respiratory conditions, such as CVA, may be more susceptible to the effects of environmental pollutants due to age-related declines in lung function, immune function, and antioxidant defenses, leading to increased susceptibility to pollutant-induced exacerbations and respiratory morbidity.
- **Occupational Exposures:** Occupational exposures to environmental pollutants, such as airborne particulates, dusts, fumes, and chemicals, can exacerbate respiratory symptoms and impair lung function in individuals with CVA working in industries with high levels of air pollution or occupational hazards.

5. Therapeutic Implications:

Management of environmental pollutants in individuals with CVA involves a combination of preventive measures, environmental controls, and pharmacological interventions aimed at reducing exposure, mitigating symptoms, and improving lung function. Strategies may include:

- **Allergen Avoidance:** Minimizing exposure to indoor allergens (e.g., dust mites, animal dander, mold) and outdoor allergens (e.g., pollen, fungal spores) through environmental controls (e.g., air filtration, mattress and pillow encasements), lifestyle modifications (e.g., pet restrictions, humidity control), and allergen immunotherapy may help reduce allergen-induced exacerbations of CVA.
- **Air Quality Monitoring:** Monitoring air quality indices (e.g., Air Quality Index [AQI], Pollutant Standards Index [PSI]) and pollutant levels (e.g., PM2.5, NO2, ozone) can help identify high-risk periods and locations for pollutant exposure, allowing individuals with CVA to take preventive measures (e.g., staying indoors, wearing respiratory masks) to reduce exposure and minimize respiratory symptoms.
- **Pharmacological Interventions:** Pharmacological interventions, including inhaled corticosteroids, bronchodilators (e.g., β2-agonists), leukotriene receptor antagonists, and biologic agents targeting inflammatory pathways (e.g., anti-IgE antibodies, anti-IL-5 antibodies), may be used to suppress airway inflammation, alleviate respiratory symptoms, and improve lung function in individuals with CVA exposed to environmental pollutants.

Conclusion:

In conclusion, environmental pollutants are significant contributors to cough-variant asthma, exacerbating airway inflammation, bronchial hyperresponsiveness, and respiratory symptoms in affected individuals. Understanding the diverse array of pollutants, their mechanisms of action, and their impact on CVA is essential for elucidating disease mechanisms, identifying exacerbating factors, and optimizing management strategies. By targeting environmental pollutants, implementing preventive measures, and adopting personalized treatment approaches tailored to individual patients' pollutant exposures and disease severity, clinicians can improve outcomes and quality of life for individuals with this distinct clinical phenotype of asthma.

Occupational Exposures and Their Impact on Cough-Variant Asthma

Occupational exposures represent a significant risk factor for respiratory diseases, including cough-variant asthma (CVA). Exposure to various occupational hazards, such as airborne particulates, dusts, fumes, gases, and chemicals, can exacerbate airway inflammation, bronchial hyperresponsiveness, and respiratory symptoms in individuals with CVA. Understanding the diverse array of occupational exposures, their mechanisms of action, and their impact on CVA is crucial for elucidating disease mechanisms, identifying exacerbating factors, and optimizing management strategies. This section explores the multifaceted relationship between occupational exposures and CVA, highlighting key occupational hazards, immune responses, and therapeutic implications.

1. Common Occupational Hazards:

Numerous occupational hazards can trigger or exacerbate respiratory symptoms in individuals with CVA. Common occupational exposures associated with CVA include:

- **Airborne Particulates:** Fine particulate matter (PM2.5) and respirable dusts generated from various industrial processes, such as mining, construction, agriculture, and manufacturing, can irritate the airways, induce airway

inflammation, and exacerbate respiratory symptoms in individuals with CVA exposed to occupational dusts.
- **Chemical Irritants:** Chemical irritants, such as volatile organic compounds (VOCs), ozone, sulfur dioxide (SO2), nitrogen dioxide (NO2), and chlorine gas, released from industrial chemicals, cleaning products, disinfectants, and solvents, can irritate the airways, induce bronchospasm, and exacerbate respiratory symptoms in individuals with CVA sensitive to chemical exposures.
- **Fumes and Gases:** Fumes and gases generated from welding, soldering, metalworking, and combustion processes can contain toxic substances, such as metal oxides, fumes, and vapors, which can trigger airway inflammation, oxidative stress, and exacerbation of respiratory symptoms in individuals with CVA exposed to occupational fumes and gases.
- **Biological Agents:** Biological agents, such as bacteria, fungi, and allergens, present in occupational settings, such as healthcare facilities, agricultural settings, and animal handling areas, can trigger allergic sensitization, induce airway inflammation, and exacerbate respiratory symptoms in individuals with CVA exposed to occupational allergens.

2. Mechanisms of Action:

Occupational exposures exert their effects on the respiratory system through multiple mechanisms, including:

- **Direct Airway Irritation:** Occupational hazards, such as airborne particulates, dusts, fumes, and chemical irritants, can directly irritate the airways, induce airway inflammation, and trigger bronchospasm in individuals with CVA sensitive to occupational exposures.
- **Airway Inflammation:** Occupational exposures can promote airway inflammation by activating

inflammatory cells (e.g., neutrophils, eosinophils), releasing pro-inflammatory cytokines (e.g., interleukin-6 [IL-6], interleukin-8 [IL-8]), and promoting oxidative stress-mediated damage to airway epithelial cells in individuals with CVA.
- **Bronchial Hyperresponsiveness:** Occupational exposures can enhance bronchial hyperresponsiveness by stimulating bronchial smooth muscle contraction, increasing airway resistance, and impairing lung function in individuals with CVA exposed to occupational hazards.
- **Immune Dysregulation:** Occupational exposures can disrupt immune responses by modulating cytokine production, impairing antigen presentation, and promoting Th2-mediated allergic inflammation in individuals with CVA exposed to occupational allergens.

3. Impact on Disease Severity:

Occupational exposures can significantly impact the severity and natural history of CVA, leading to exacerbations, worsening of respiratory symptoms, and impaired lung function in affected individuals. Long-term exposure to high levels of occupational hazards, such as dusts, fumes, and chemical irritants, is associated with increased risk of asthma development, progression, and poor treatment outcomes in individuals with CVA. Occupational-induced exacerbations of CVA are characterized by increased coughing episodes, wheezing, dyspnea, and reduced quality of life, necessitating prompt identification and mitigation of occupational exposures to improve disease control and outcomes.

4. Vulnerable Populations:

Certain populations may be particularly susceptible to the adverse effects of occupational exposures on CVA, including:

- **Workers in High-Risk Industries:** Individuals working in industries with high levels of occupational hazards, such as construction, mining, manufacturing, agriculture, healthcare, and cleaning services, may be at increased risk of developing CVA due to chronic exposure to airborne particulates, dusts, fumes, and chemicals.
- **Sensitized Individuals:** Individuals with pre-existing sensitization to occupational allergens, such as healthcare workers exposed to latex allergens, laboratory workers exposed to animal dander, and agricultural workers exposed to plant allergens, may be more susceptible to the effects of occupational exposures on CVA, leading to exacerbation of respiratory symptoms and impaired lung function.
- **Smokers:** Smokers with CVA may be at increased risk of occupational exacerbations due to the combined effects of tobacco smoke exposure and occupational hazards on airway inflammation, bronchial hyperresponsiveness, and respiratory symptoms.

5. Therapeutic Implications:

Management of occupational exposures in individuals with CVA involves a combination of preventive measures, environmental controls, and pharmacological interventions aimed at reducing exposure, mitigating symptoms, and improving lung function. Strategies may include:

- **Workplace Hazard Controls:** Implementing engineering controls (e.g., ventilation systems, dust extraction systems), administrative controls (e.g., work practices, training programs), and personal protective equipment (e.g., respiratory masks, gloves) can help minimize occupational exposures and reduce the risk of respiratory symptoms in individuals with CVA working in high-risk industries.

- **Allergen Avoidance:** Minimizing exposure to occupational allergens (e.g., latex, animal dander, plant allergens) through environmental controls (e.g., allergen-free workspaces, personal protective equipment), allergen monitoring, and allergen immunotherapy may help reduce allergic sensitization and prevent exacerbation of respiratory symptoms in sensitized individuals with CVA.
- **Pharmacological Interventions:** Pharmacological interventions, including inhaled corticosteroids, bronchodilators (e.g., β2-agonists), leukotriene receptor antagonists, and biologic agents targeting inflammatory pathways (e.g., anti-IgE antibodies, anti-IL-5 antibodies), may be used to suppress airway inflammation, alleviate respiratory symptoms, and improve lung function in individuals with CVA exposed to occupational hazards.

Conclusion:

In conclusion, occupational exposures are significant risk factors for cough-variant asthma, exacerbating airway inflammation, bronchial hyperresponsiveness, and respiratory symptoms in affected individuals. Understanding the diverse array of occupational hazards, their mechanisms of action, and their impact on CVA is essential for elucidating disease mechanisms, identifying exacerbating factors, and optimizing management strategies. By targeting occupational exposures, implementing preventive measures, and adopting personalized treatment approaches tailored to individual patients' occupational hazards and disease severity, clinicians can improve outcomes and quality of life for individuals with this distinct clinical phenotype of asthma.

Exercise-Induced Asthma and its Relation to Cough-Variant

Asthma

Exercise-induced asthma (EIA), also known as exercise-induced bronchoconstriction (EIB), is a common phenomenon characterized by the transient narrowing of airways during or after physical exertion. While it shares similarities with cough-variant asthma (CVA), it presents unique challenges in diagnosis, management, and understanding its pathophysiology. This section delves into the complexities of EIA, its relationship with CVA, and strategies for effective management.

1. Definition and Characteristics:

Exercise-induced asthma refers to the occurrence of asthma symptoms, such as coughing, wheezing, chest tightness, and shortness of breath, triggered by physical activity. Unlike typical asthma, where symptoms may be persistent or triggered by various stimuli, EIA specifically occurs during or shortly after exercise. It can affect individuals of all ages, including children and adults, and may occur in those with or without a history of asthma.

2. Pathophysiology:

The exact mechanisms underlying EIA are not fully understood, but it is believed to involve a combination of airway dehydration, cooling of airways, increased ventilation, and release of inflammatory mediators. During exercise, individuals breathe rapidly through their mouths, leading to the loss of water and heat from the airways, which can cause airway dehydration and cooling. This process may trigger the release of inflammatory mediators, such as histamine, leukotrienes, and prostaglandins, leading to airway smooth muscle contraction and bronchoconstriction.

3. Relationship with Cough-Variant Asthma:

While EIA and CVA are distinct clinical entities, they often coexist or overlap in individuals with asthma. Some individuals with CVA may experience coughing or other respiratory symptoms triggered by exercise, leading to a diagnosis of both CVA and EIA. Conversely, individuals with EIA may also experience coughing as a predominant symptom, mimicking the presentation of CVA. The coexistence of EIA and CVA highlights the heterogeneity of asthma phenotypes and underscores the importance of comprehensive evaluation and individualized management approaches.

4. Diagnosis:

Diagnosing EIA involves assessing symptoms, spirometry before and after exercise challenge, and/or measuring peak expiratory flow rates before and after exercise. Exercise challenge testing, such as a treadmill or cycle ergometer test, can reproduce symptoms in a controlled environment and help confirm the diagnosis. Additionally, ruling out other conditions that may mimic EIA, such as vocal cord dysfunction or cardiac conditions, is essential for accurate diagnosis.

5. Management Strategies:

Management of EIA focuses on both pharmacological and non-pharmacological approaches aimed at preventing symptoms and optimizing exercise tolerance:

- **Pharmacological Interventions:** Short-acting beta-agonists (SABAs), such as albuterol, are commonly used as pre-exercise bronchodilators to prevent or reduce symptoms of EIA. Inhaled corticosteroids (ICS) may be used as maintenance therapy for individuals with persistent EIA or those with coexisting asthma. Additionally, leukotriene receptor antagonists, such as montelukast, may be effective in some individuals, particularly those with allergic asthma.

- **Non-pharmacological Interventions:** Warm-up exercises before strenuous activity, gradual intensity progression during exercise, and wearing a face mask or scarf during exercise in cold or dry environments can help reduce the severity of EIA symptoms. Avoiding triggers, such as exposure to allergens or pollutants during exercise, and maintaining optimal asthma control through regular monitoring and adherence to controller medications are essential components of EIA management.

6. Prognosis and Outlook:

With appropriate management and adherence to treatment strategies, most individuals with EIA can participate in regular physical activity and sports without significant limitations. However, EIA symptoms may persist or worsen if left untreated, leading to decreased exercise tolerance, reduced quality of life, and increased risk of asthma exacerbations. Regular follow-up visits with healthcare providers, monitoring of symptoms and lung function, and adjustments to treatment regimens as needed are essential for achieving optimal outcomes in individuals with EIA.

Conclusion:

Exercise-induced asthma is a common phenomenon characterized by the onset of asthma symptoms during or after physical exertion. While it shares similarities with cough-variant asthma, it presents unique challenges in diagnosis and management. Understanding the pathophysiology, relationship with cough-variant asthma, and effective management strategies for exercise-induced asthma is essential for optimizing outcomes and quality of life in affected individuals. By implementing comprehensive evaluation, individualized treatment approaches, and preventive measures, clinicians can help individuals with exercise-induced asthma achieve symptom control, maintain optimal exercise tolerance, and lead active, healthy lives.

Gastroesophageal Reflux Disease (GERD) and its Association with Cough-Variant Asthma

Gastroesophageal reflux disease (GERD) is a chronic condition characterized by the retrograde flow of gastric contents into the esophagus, leading to symptoms such as heartburn, regurgitation, and chest discomfort. While GERD primarily affects the gastrointestinal tract, it can also manifest with extraesophageal symptoms, including coughing, throat clearing, and wheezing. This section explores the complex relationship between GERD and cough-variant asthma (CVA), highlighting the mechanisms, clinical manifestations, diagnostic considerations, and management strategies for individuals with both conditions.

1. Pathophysiology:

GERD-related cough is thought to occur due to microaspiration of gastric contents into the airways, leading to irritation and inflammation of the larynx, trachea, and bronchi. Acidic refluxate can activate sensory receptors in the distal esophagus and airways, triggering cough reflexes and exacerbating respiratory symptoms in susceptible individuals. Additionally, the presence of esophageal dysmotility, impaired esophageal clearance, and altered cough reflex sensitivity may further contribute to GERD-related cough in some individuals.

2. Clinical Manifestations:

GERD-related cough often presents as a non-productive, chronic cough that worsens after eating, lying down, or during periods of increased intra-abdominal pressure. The cough may be dry or accompanied by minimal sputum production and may persist despite treatment with cough suppressants or bronchodilators. Individuals with GERD-related cough may also experience symptoms of heartburn, regurgitation, dysphagia, or throat discomfort, which can help distinguish GERD-related cough from other causes of chronic cough, including CVA.

3. Diagnostic Considerations:

Diagnosing GERD-related cough requires a comprehensive evaluation, including a detailed medical history, physical examination, and diagnostic testing. Endoscopic evaluation with esophageal pH monitoring or impedance testing can confirm the presence of GERD and assess the extent of esophageal acid exposure. High-resolution esophageal manometry may help identify esophageal dysmotility or impaired esophageal clearance, which can contribute to GERD-related cough. Additionally, chest imaging studies, such as chest X-rays or computed tomography (CT) scans, may be indicated to rule out other respiratory conditions or complications of GERD.

4. Association with Cough-Variant Asthma:

GERD and cough-variant asthma frequently coexist or overlap in individuals with chronic cough, making it challenging to differentiate between the two conditions based solely on clinical presentation. While cough-variant asthma primarily involves airway inflammation and bronchial hyperresponsiveness, GERD-related cough may exacerbate respiratory symptoms and mimic the presentation of cough-variant asthma. The coexistence of GERD and cough-variant asthma underscores the importance of comprehensive evaluation and individualized treatment approaches for individuals with chronic cough and respiratory symptoms.

5. Management Strategies:

Management of GERD-related cough involves a combination of

lifestyle modifications, pharmacological interventions, and, in some cases, surgical or endoscopic procedures aimed at reducing acid reflux, controlling symptoms, and improving quality of life:

- **Lifestyle Modifications:** Avoiding trigger foods (e.g., spicy foods, caffeine, alcohol), maintaining a healthy weight, elevating the head of the bed, and avoiding lying down immediately after eating can help reduce acid reflux and alleviate symptoms of GERD-related cough.
- **Pharmacological Interventions:** Proton pump inhibitors (PPIs), histamine H2-receptor antagonists, and prokinetic agents may be prescribed to suppress gastric acid secretion, promote esophageal healing, and improve esophageal motility in individuals with GERD-related cough. Antacids or alginate-based formulations may provide symptomatic relief of heartburn and regurgitation.
- **Surgical or Endoscopic Procedures:** In individuals with refractory GERD or complications such as Barrett's esophagus or esophageal strictures, surgical interventions, such as fundoplication or endoscopic therapies (e.g., radiofrequency ablation, endoscopic mucosal resection), may be considered to reduce acid reflux and prevent long-term complications.

6. Prognosis and Outlook:

With appropriate management and adherence to treatment strategies, most individuals with GERD-related cough can achieve symptom control, improve cough resolution, and reduce the frequency and severity of coughing episodes. However, GERD-related cough may persist or recur if left untreated or inadequately managed, leading to decreased quality of life and impaired respiratory function. Regular follow-up visits with healthcare providers, monitoring of symptoms, and adjustments to treatment regimens as needed are essential for optimizing outcomes in individuals with GERD-related cough.

Conclusion:

Gastroesophageal reflux disease (GERD) is a common condition characterized by the retrograde flow of gastric contents into the esophagus, leading to symptoms such as heartburn, regurgitation, and chest discomfort. GERD-related cough, a common extraesophageal manifestation of GERD, can mimic the presentation of cough-variant asthma (CVA) and contribute to chronic cough and respiratory symptoms in affected individuals. Understanding the complex relationship between GERD and CVA, evaluating for both conditions in individuals with chronic cough, and implementing comprehensive treatment approaches tailored to individual patient needs are essential for achieving optimal outcomes and improving quality of life in individuals with GERD-related cough and coexisting respiratory conditions.

Psychological Stress and its Impact on Cough-Variant Asthma

Psychological stress is a complex phenomenon that can influence various aspects of health, including respiratory conditions such as cough-variant asthma (CVA). Stress encompasses a wide range of psychological and physiological responses to perceived threats or challenges, and its effects on the immune system, inflammatory pathways, and respiratory function are well-documented. This section explores the relationship between psychological stress and CVA, highlighting the mechanisms, clinical manifestations, diagnostic considerations, and management strategies for individuals affected by both conditions.

1. Mechanisms of Action:

Psychological stress can influence the pathogenesis and clinical course of CVA through multiple mechanisms, including:

- **Neuroendocrine Responses:** Stress activates the hypothalamic-pituitary-adrenal (HPA) axis and the sympathetic-adrenal-medullary (SAM) axis, leading to the release of stress hormones such as cortisol and adrenaline. These hormones can modulate immune responses, inflammatory pathways, and bronchial smooth muscle tone, potentially exacerbating airway inflammation and bronchial hyperresponsiveness in individuals with CVA.
- **Immune Dysregulation:** Chronic stress can dysregulate immune responses, leading to alterations in cytokine production, immune cell trafficking, and inflammatory signaling pathways. Stress-induced immune dysregulation may promote airway inflammation, allergic sensitization, and exacerbation of respiratory symptoms in individuals with CVA, particularly those with comorbid allergic conditions.
- **Autonomic Nervous System Dysfunction:** Stress can alter autonomic nervous system function, leading to sympathetic nervous system activation and parasympathetic withdrawal. These autonomic changes may increase airway smooth muscle tone, enhance bronchial reactivity, and exacerbate respiratory symptoms in individuals with CVA, particularly during periods of heightened stress or emotional arousal.

2. Clinical Manifestations:

Psychological stress can manifest with a wide range of respiratory symptoms in individuals with CVA, including:

- **Increased Coughing Episodes:** Stress-induced changes in airway reactivity and cough reflex sensitivity may

lead to an increase in coughing episodes in individuals with CVA, particularly during periods of acute stress or emotional distress.
- **Worsening of Respiratory Symptoms:** Stress-related exacerbations of CVA may manifest with worsening of respiratory symptoms, such as wheezing, dyspnea, and chest tightness, which can mimic asthma exacerbations triggered by other factors.
- **Impaired Disease Control:** Chronic stress may interfere with asthma management strategies, medication adherence, and self-care behaviors, leading to suboptimal disease control and increased risk of asthma exacerbations in affected individuals.

3. Diagnostic Considerations:

Assessing the impact of psychological stress on CVA requires a comprehensive evaluation, including a detailed medical history, assessment of psychosocial factors, and consideration of stress-related triggers or exacerbating factors. Screening tools, such as standardized questionnaires or scales assessing stress, anxiety, and depression, may help identify individuals at risk of stress-related exacerbations of CVA. Collaborative assessment by healthcare providers, including pulmonologists, allergists, and mental health professionals, can facilitate comprehensive evaluation and management of stress-related respiratory symptoms in individuals with CVA.

4. Management Strategies:

Management of stress-related exacerbations of CVA involves a combination of pharmacological and non-pharmacological interventions aimed at reducing stress levels, alleviating respiratory symptoms, and improving disease control:
- **Stress Management Techniques:** Stress reduction techniques, such as relaxation exercises, deep breathing

exercises, mindfulness meditation, and cognitive-behavioral therapy (CBT), can help individuals with CVA cope with stress, manage anxiety, and reduce the frequency and severity of stress-related respiratory symptoms.
- **Behavioral Interventions:** Adopting healthy lifestyle behaviors, such as regular exercise, adequate sleep, balanced nutrition, and social support, can help mitigate the impact of stress on respiratory function and improve overall well-being in individuals with CVA.
- **Pharmacological Interventions:** In some cases, pharmacological interventions, such as anxiolytics, antidepressants, or stress-relieving medications, may be prescribed to alleviate symptoms of anxiety or depression and improve stress-related respiratory symptoms in individuals with CVA.

5. Prognosis and Outlook:

With appropriate management and support, most individuals with stress-related exacerbations of CVA can achieve symptom control, improve disease management, and reduce the impact of stress on respiratory function and quality of life. However, stress-related respiratory symptoms may persist or recur if underlying stressors are not addressed or if individuals experience ongoing stressors or psychological distress. Regular follow-up visits with healthcare providers, monitoring of stress levels and respiratory symptoms, and adjustments to treatment regimens as needed are essential for optimizing outcomes and improving quality of life in individuals with stress-related respiratory conditions.

Conclusion:

Psychological stress can significantly impact the pathogenesis and clinical course of cough-variant asthma (CVA), leading to exacerbations, worsening of respiratory symptoms, and impaired disease control in affected individuals. Understanding the mechanisms underlying stress-related exacerbations of CVA, assessing psychosocial factors, and implementing comprehensive management strategies aimed at reducing stress levels, alleviating respiratory symptoms, and improving disease control are essential for optimizing outcomes and improving quality of life in individuals with stress-related respiratory conditions. By addressing psychological stress as a modifiable risk factor and integrating stress management techniques into asthma management plans, healthcare providers can help individuals with CVA achieve symptom control, reduce exacerbations, and lead fulfilling, healthy lives.

CHAPTER 4: CLINICAL EVALUATION AND DIAGNOSTIC APPROACH

Patient History and Symptom Assessment in Cough-Variant Asthma

Obtaining a thorough patient history and conducting a comprehensive symptom assessment are essential components of diagnosing and managing cough-variant asthma (CVA). Since cough is the predominant symptom in CVA, understanding the nature, duration, triggers, and associated symptoms of cough is crucial for accurate diagnosis and personalized treatment planning. This section outlines the key elements of patient history and symptom assessment in individuals suspected of having CVA.

1. Initial Patient Evaluation:

- **Chief Complaint:** Begin by identifying the patient's chief complaint, which is typically chronic cough in the case of CVA. Encourage the patient to describe the

characteristics of their cough, including its frequency, duration, severity, and any associated symptoms.
- **Medical History:** Obtain a detailed medical history, including past medical conditions, respiratory illnesses, allergies, environmental exposures, medication use, and family history of asthma or allergic conditions. Pay particular attention to any history of atopic diseases, such as allergic rhinitis or eczema, as they are commonly associated with CVA.
- **Risk Factors:** Assess for potential risk factors associated with CVA, such as exposure to environmental pollutants, occupational hazards, tobacco smoke, respiratory infections, or psychological stressors. Inquire about any recent changes in the patient's environment or lifestyle that may have triggered or exacerbated their cough.

2. Symptom Assessment:

- **Cough Characteristics:** Inquire about the nature of the cough, including its timing (daytime vs. nighttime), frequency (intermittent vs. persistent), duration (acute vs. chronic), and productivity (dry vs. productive). Determine whether the cough is triggered or worsened by specific factors, such as exposure to allergens, cold air, exercise, laughter, or respiratory infections.
- **Associated Symptoms:** Evaluate for any associated respiratory symptoms, such as wheezing, dyspnea, chest tightness, or sputum production, which may suggest underlying airway inflammation or bronchial hyperresponsiveness. Inquire about symptoms of allergic rhinitis, such as nasal congestion, sneezing, or postnasal drip, as they often coexist with CVA.
- **Exacerbating Factors:** Identify potential triggers or exacerbating factors that worsen the patient's cough, such as exposure to allergens (e.g., pollen, dust mites, pet dander), respiratory irritants (e.g., smoke, pollution,

strong odors), cold air, exercise, stress, or respiratory infections. Determine whether the cough improves with rest or during vacations away from home.

3. Review of Systems:

- **Respiratory System:** Conduct a systematic review of respiratory symptoms, including cough, wheezing, dyspnea, chest pain, or nocturnal awakenings due to coughing or respiratory distress. Inquire about any history of recurrent respiratory infections, sinusitis, or gastroesophageal reflux disease (GERD) symptoms, as they may be associated with CVA.
- **Allergic Symptoms:** Assess for symptoms of allergic rhinitis, such as nasal congestion, sneezing, itching, or postnasal drip, which often coexist with CVA and may contribute to cough exacerbations.
- **Gastrointestinal Symptoms:** Inquire about symptoms of GERD, such as heartburn, regurgitation, dysphagia, or throat discomfort, as GERD-related cough is a common differential diagnosis for CVA.

4. Psychological Assessment:

- **Stress and Anxiety:** Assess for symptoms of psychological stress, anxiety, or depression, as psychological factors can influence cough severity and perception in individuals with CVA. Inquire about recent life stressors, emotional distress, or changes in mood or mental health that may be contributing to the patient's cough.

5. Differential Diagnosis Considerations:

- **Asthma Phenotypes:** Consider other asthma phenotypes that may present with cough as a predominant symptom, such as classic asthma, eosinophilic asthma, or aspirin-

exacerbated respiratory disease (AERD). Evaluate for features suggestive of these phenotypes, such as bronchial hyperresponsiveness, sputum eosinophilia, or aspirin sensitivity.
- **Other Respiratory Conditions:** Rule out other respiratory conditions that may mimic CVA, such as upper airway cough syndrome (UACS), postnasal drip syndrome, gastroesophageal reflux disease (GERD), or non-asthmatic eosinophilic bronchitis. Conduct appropriate diagnostic tests, such as spirometry, bronchial provocation testing, sputum analysis, or laryngoscopy, as indicated.

Conclusion:

Patient history and symptom assessment are critical components of diagnosing cough-variant asthma (CVA) and differentiating it from other respiratory conditions presenting with chronic cough. By obtaining a detailed medical history, conducting a comprehensive symptom assessment, and considering potential triggers, exacerbating factors, and differential diagnoses, healthcare providers can accurately diagnose CVA and develop personalized treatment plans tailored to individual patient needs. A multidisciplinary approach, involving collaboration between pulmonologists, allergists, otolaryngologists, and mental health professionals, may be necessary for comprehensive evaluation and management of CVA and associated comorbidities.

Physical Examination Findings in Cough-Variant Asthma

A thorough physical examination plays a crucial role in the evaluation of individuals suspected of having cough-variant asthma (CVA). While cough is the primary symptom in CVA, certain physical examination findings may provide valuable clues to support the diagnosis, assess disease severity, and identify potential complications or comorbidities. This section outlines the key physical examination findings that healthcare providers should assess when evaluating individuals with suspected CVA.

1. General Appearance:

- **Respiratory Distress:** Evaluate for signs of respiratory distress, such as increased respiratory rate, use of accessory muscles, nasal flaring, or paradoxical chest wall movement, which may suggest underlying airway obstruction or bronchospasm.
- **Nutritional Status:** Assess the patient's nutritional status and overall health, as poor nutrition or weight loss may indicate underlying disease severity or complications of chronic cough.

2. Vital Signs:

- **Respiratory Rate:** Measure the patient's respiratory rate at rest and during periods of activity to assess for tachypnea, which may indicate increased work of breathing or respiratory compromise.
- **Heart Rate:** Assess the patient's heart rate for signs of tachycardia, which may occur in response to bronchospasm, hypoxia, or anxiety associated with coughing episodes.
- **Blood Pressure:** Measure the patient's blood pressure to assess for hypertension, which may be associated with underlying stress or anxiety exacerbating cough symptoms.

3. Head and Neck Examination:

- **Nasal Examination:** Evaluate the nasal passages for

signs of congestion, discharge, or allergic rhinitis, which may suggest upper airway inflammation or postnasal drip contributing to cough symptoms.
- **Oropharyngeal Examination:** Inspect the oropharynx for signs of inflammation, erythema, or postnasal drip, which may indicate upper airway irritation or GERD-related cough.

4. Chest Examination:

- **Lung Auscultation:** Auscultate the lungs bilaterally for breath sounds, wheezes, crackles, or diminished breath sounds, which may indicate underlying airway obstruction, bronchospasm, or consolidation.
- **Percussion:** Percuss the chest wall to assess for dullness or hyperresonance, which may suggest underlying lung consolidation or air trapping.

5. Cardiovascular Examination:

- **Heart Sounds:** Listen to the heart sounds for evidence of cardiac abnormalities, such as murmurs or gallops, which may indicate underlying cardiovascular disease exacerbating cough symptoms.

6. Abdominal Examination:

- **Abdominal Palpation:** Palpate the abdomen for tenderness, distension, or organomegaly, which may suggest underlying gastrointestinal conditions, such as GERD or abdominal distension exacerbating cough symptoms.

7. Neurological Examination:

- **Mental Status:** Assess the patient's mental status and cognitive function for signs of anxiety, depression, or cognitive impairment, which may influence cough perception and management strategies.

8. Skin Examination:

- **Allergic Skin Manifestations:** Inspect the skin for signs of allergic dermatitis, urticaria, or eczema, which may indicate underlying atopic conditions predisposing to CVA.

Conclusion:

A comprehensive physical examination is essential for evaluating individuals suspected of having cough-variant asthma (CVA) and assessing disease severity, complications, or comorbidities. By systematically assessing vital signs, general appearance, head and neck, chest, cardiovascular, abdominal, neurological, and skin findings, healthcare providers can gather valuable clinical information to support the diagnosis of CVA and guide treatment decisions. Additionally, identifying potential triggers, exacerbating factors, and associated comorbidities through physical examination findings can help inform a multidisciplinary approach to the management of CVA and improve outcomes for affected individuals.

Pulmonary Function Tests in Cough-Variant Asthma

Pulmonary function tests (PFTs) play a vital role in the diagnosis, assessment, and management of cough-variant asthma (CVA). These tests provide objective measures of lung function, airway responsiveness, and bronchodilator response, helping healthcare providers evaluate the severity of airway obstruction, identify reversible airflow limitation, and monitor treatment response in individuals with CVA. This section explores the different types of PFTs commonly used in the evaluation of CVA, their interpretation, and their clinical significance.

1. Spirometry:

Spirometry is the most commonly performed pulmonary function test and serves as the cornerstone of lung function assessment in individuals with CVA. It measures the volume and flow rates of air that can be forcefully exhaled from the lungs after a maximal inhalation. Key spirometric parameters include:

- **Forced Vital Capacity (FVC):** The total volume of air exhaled forcefully and maximally from full inspiration to maximal expiration.
- **Forced Expiratory Volume in 1 second (FEV1):** The volume of air forcefully exhaled during the first second of the FVC maneuver.
- **FEV1/FVC Ratio:** The ratio of FEV1 to FVC, expressed as a percentage. A reduced FEV1/FVC ratio suggests airflow obstruction, which may be indicative of asthma or other obstructive lung diseases.
- **Peak Expiratory Flow (PEF):** The maximum flow rate achieved during a forced exhalation effort, measured in liters per minute. PEF monitoring may be used for assessing airflow limitation and monitoring asthma control over time.

2. Bronchodilator Response Testing:

Bronchodilator response testing is often performed following baseline spirometry to assess for reversibility of airflow limitation, which is characteristic of asthma. After baseline spirometry, a short-acting bronchodilator, typically albuterol, is administered via inhalation, and spirometry is repeated after a specified period (usually 15-30 minutes) to assess for changes in lung function. A significant bronchodilator response is defined as an increase in FEV1 of ≥12% and ≥200 mL from baseline.

3. Methacholine Challenge Test:

The methacholine challenge test is used to assess airway hyperresponsiveness, a hallmark feature of asthma, in individuals with suspected CVA who have normal baseline spirometry. During the test, increasing concentrations of methacholine, a bronchoconstrictor, are inhaled via nebulization, and spirometry is performed at regular intervals to measure changes in lung function. A positive test result is defined as a ≥20% decrease in FEV1 from baseline at a specified concentration of methacholine.

4. Fractional Exhaled Nitric Oxide (FeNO) Measurement:

FeNO measurement is a non-invasive test that assesses airway inflammation, particularly eosinophilic inflammation, which is commonly associated with asthma. FeNO levels reflect the concentration of nitric oxide (NO) in exhaled breath and are measured using a portable analyzer. Elevated FeNO levels (>25-50 ppb) may suggest underlying airway inflammation and eosinophilic asthma phenotypes, including CVA.

5. Interpretation and Clinical Significance:

Interpretation of PFT results in individuals with CVA requires careful consideration of clinical context, patient symptoms, and other diagnostic findings. Key considerations include:

- **Airflow Limitation:** Reduced FEV1/FVC ratio and/or FEV1 may indicate airflow limitation suggestive of asthma or obstructive lung disease, particularly if accompanied by a significant bronchodilator response.
- **Airway Hyperresponsiveness:** A positive methacholine challenge test or increased FeNO levels may support the diagnosis of airway hyperresponsiveness and asthma in individuals with suspected CVA, particularly in those with normal baseline spirometry.

- **Treatment Monitoring:** Serial PFTs can be used to monitor treatment response, assess disease progression, and guide adjustments to asthma management strategies in individuals with CVA. Improvements in FEV1, FEV1/FVC ratio, and PEF following bronchodilator administration may indicate effective bronchodilator therapy and asthma control.

Conclusion:

Pulmonary function tests are valuable diagnostic tools in the evaluation of cough-variant asthma, providing objective measures of lung function, airway responsiveness, and inflammation. Spirometry, bronchodilator response testing, methacholine challenge testing, and FeNO measurement play complementary roles in confirming the diagnosis, assessing disease severity, and monitoring treatment response in individuals with CVA. Interpretation of PFT results requires careful consideration of clinical context, patient symptoms, and other diagnostic findings to guide individualized management strategies and optimize outcomes for individuals with CVA. By incorporating PFTs into the diagnostic algorithm for CVA, healthcare providers can enhance diagnostic accuracy, tailor treatment regimens, and improve patient care in this distinct clinical phenotype of asthma.

The Methacholine Challenge Test: A Diagnostic Tool for Cough-Variant Asthma

The methacholine challenge test (MCT) serves as a valuable diagnostic tool in the evaluation of cough-variant asthma (CVA), providing insights into airway hyperresponsiveness, a hallmark feature of asthma. This test involves the inhalation of increasing concentrations of methacholine, a cholinergic agonist that induces bronchoconstriction, followed by spirometric measurements to assess changes in lung function. This section delves into the principles, methodology, interpretation, and clinical significance of the methacholine challenge test in the diagnosis and management of CVA.

1. Principles of the Methacholine Challenge Test:

The methacholine challenge test is based on the principle of inducing bronchoconstriction in individuals with airway hyperresponsiveness, a characteristic feature of asthma. Methacholine acts as a cholinergic agonist, stimulating muscarinic receptors on airway smooth muscle cells and leading to bronchoconstriction and airway narrowing. In individuals with asthma, even small doses of methacholine can trigger exaggerated bronchoconstriction due to underlying airway inflammation and increased bronchial reactivity.

2. Methodology of the Methacholine Challenge Test:

The methacholine challenge test is typically performed in a specialized pulmonary function laboratory under the supervision of trained healthcare professionals. The test involves the following steps:

- **Baseline Spirometry:** Baseline spirometry is performed to assess the patient's lung function before methacholine administration. Key spirometric parameters, including forced expiratory volume in 1 second (FEV1) and forced vital capacity (FVC), are measured to establish baseline lung function.
- **Methacholine Inhalation:** Increasing concentrations of methacholine are administered via nebulization, typically starting with a low concentration and escalating in a stepwise fashion until a predetermined endpoint is reached. Methacholine solutions are aerosolized using a nebulizer and delivered to the patient

via a mouthpiece or face mask connected to a spirometer.
- **Spirometric Measurements:** Spirometry is performed at regular intervals (usually every 1-3 minutes) following each methacholine inhalation to assess changes in lung function. Spirometric parameters, including FEV1 and FVC, are measured and recorded after each methacholine dose to monitor for airway narrowing and bronchoconstriction.
- **Test Termination:** The methacholine challenge test is terminated when a predetermined endpoint is reached, such as a significant decrease in FEV1 from baseline or a maximum methacholine dose. A positive test result is typically defined as a ≥20% decrease in FEV1 from baseline at a specified concentration of methacholine.

3. Interpretation of Methacholine Challenge Test Results:

Interpretation of methacholine challenge test results requires careful consideration of clinical context, patient symptoms, and other diagnostic findings. Key considerations include:

- **Airway Hyperresponsiveness:** A positive methacholine challenge test, characterized by a significant decrease in FEV1 from baseline at a specified concentration of methacholine, suggests the presence of airway hyperresponsiveness and increased bronchial reactivity, which are characteristic features of asthma.
- **Sensitivity and Specificity:** The sensitivity and specificity of the methacholine challenge test vary depending on the cutoff criteria used to define a positive test result and the population being tested. While the test is highly sensitive for detecting airway hyperresponsiveness in individuals with asthma, false-positive results may occur in individuals without asthma, particularly in those with other respiratory conditions or comorbidities.

- **Clinical Correlation:** Methacholine challenge test results should be interpreted in conjunction with the patient's clinical history, symptoms, and other diagnostic findings to confirm the diagnosis of CVA and guide treatment decisions. Positive test results in the absence of typical asthma symptoms or other supportive evidence should prompt further evaluation to rule out alternative diagnoses.

4. Clinical Significance of the Methacholine Challenge Test:

The methacholine challenge test plays a crucial role in the diagnosis and management of cough-variant asthma, providing objective evidence of airway hyperresponsiveness and increased bronchial reactivity. Key clinical applications of the methacholine challenge test in CVA include:

- **Confirming the Diagnosis:** A positive methacholine challenge test confirms the diagnosis of asthma in individuals with suspected CVA who have normal baseline spirometry and helps differentiate CVA from other causes of chronic cough.
- **Assessing Disease Severity:** The degree of bronchoconstriction induced by methacholine inhalation can provide insights into the severity of airway hyperresponsiveness and guide treatment decisions in individuals with CVA.
- **Monitoring Treatment Response:** Serial methacholine challenge tests can be used to monitor treatment response, assess disease progression, and guide adjustments to asthma management strategies in individuals with CVA. Improvements in airway hyperresponsiveness following treatment may indicate effective asthma control and guide treatment decisions.

Conclusion:

The methacholine challenge test serves as a valuable diagnostic tool in the evaluation of cough-variant asthma, providing objective evidence of airway hyperresponsiveness and increased bronchial reactivity. By inducing bronchoconstriction in response to methacholine inhalation, the test helps confirm the diagnosis of asthma, assess disease severity, and monitor treatment response in individuals with CVA. Interpretation of methacholine challenge test results requires careful consideration of clinical context, patient symptoms, and other diagnostic findings to guide individualized management strategies and optimize outcomes for individuals with CVA. Incorporating the methacholine challenge test into the diagnostic algorithm for CVA enhances diagnostic accuracy, facilitates early intervention, and improves patient care in this distinct clinical phenotype of asthma.

Exhaled Nitric Oxide Measurement in Cough-Variant Asthma

Exhaled nitric oxide (FeNO) measurement has emerged as a valuable non-invasive tool for assessing airway inflammation, particularly eosinophilic inflammation, in individuals with respiratory conditions such as cough-variant asthma (CVA). FeNO measurement provides quantitative information about airway inflammation, aids in the diagnosis and monitoring of asthma, and guides treatment decisions. This section explores the principles, methodology, interpretation, and clinical significance of FeNO measurement in the evaluation and management of CVA.

1. Principles of Exhaled Nitric Oxide Measurement:

Nitric oxide (NO) is a gaseous molecule produced endogenously by various cell types in the respiratory tract, including epithelial cells, macrophages, and eosinophils. In individuals with asthma, airway inflammation leads to increased production of NO by inducible nitric oxide synthase (iNOS) in response to inflammatory stimuli. FeNO measurement quantifies the concentration of NO in exhaled breath, providing a surrogate marker of airway inflammation, particularly eosinophilic inflammation, which is a characteristic feature of asthma.

2. Methodology of Exhaled Nitric Oxide Measurement:

FeNO measurement is typically performed using a portable, non-invasive device known as a nitric oxide analyzer. The test is performed in a quiet, non-contaminated environment, with the patient seated comfortably and breathing through a mouthpiece connected to the analyzer. The following steps outline the methodology of FeNO measurement:

- **Baseline Measurement:** The patient performs tidal breathing through the mouthpiece for a brief period (usually 10-15 seconds) to establish a baseline FeNO level.
- **Exhalation Maneuver:** The patient then performs a slow, steady exhalation, aiming for a flow rate of 50-100 mL/s, to collect exhaled breath into the analyzer. The exhalation maneuver is repeated multiple times to ensure reproducibility of results.
- **FeNO Measurement:** The nitric oxide analyzer quantifies the concentration of NO in parts per billion (ppb) in the exhaled breath sample. FeNO levels are typically reported as a single value or as the mean of multiple measurements.

3. Interpretation of Exhaled Nitric Oxide Measurement:

Interpretation of FeNO measurement results requires consideration of various factors, including clinical context, patient demographics, and other diagnostic findings. Key considerations include:

- **Elevated FeNO Levels:** Increased FeNO levels (>25-50 ppb) are suggestive of underlying airway inflammation, particularly eosinophilic inflammation, which is commonly associated with asthma. Elevated FeNO levels may support the diagnosis of asthma, including CVA, and guide treatment decisions.
- **Clinical Correlation:** FeNO measurement results should be interpreted in conjunction with the patient's clinical history, symptoms, and other diagnostic findings to confirm the diagnosis of CVA and guide treatment decisions. Elevated FeNO levels in the absence of typical asthma symptoms or other supportive evidence may warrant further evaluation to rule out alternative diagnoses.
- **Treatment Monitoring:** Serial FeNO measurements can be used to monitor treatment response, assess disease activity, and guide adjustments to asthma management strategies in individuals with CVA. Reductions in FeNO levels following treatment may indicate effective suppression of airway inflammation and improved asthma control.

4. Clinical Significance of Exhaled Nitric Oxide Measurement:

FeNO measurement has several clinical applications in the evaluation and management of CVA, including:

- **Diagnosis:** Elevated FeNO levels may support the diagnosis of CVA and provide additional evidence of airway inflammation, particularly in individuals with normal baseline spirometry and suspected asthma.
- **Assessment of Airway Inflammation:** FeNO measurement provides quantitative information about airway inflammation and aids in assessing the degree of eosinophilic inflammation, which is a key determinant of asthma severity and treatment response.

- **Treatment Guidance:** FeNO measurement can help guide treatment decisions by monitoring airway inflammation, assessing treatment response, and optimizing asthma management strategies in individuals with CVA. Targeted therapies aimed at reducing airway inflammation, such as inhaled corticosteroids (ICS), may be initiated or adjusted based on FeNO levels.

Conclusion:

Exhaled nitric oxide measurement is a valuable non-invasive tool for assessing airway inflammation and guiding treatment decisions in individuals with cough-variant asthma. By quantifying the concentration of nitric oxide in exhaled breath, FeNO measurement provides insights into eosinophilic inflammation, a characteristic feature of asthma, and aids in the diagnosis, monitoring, and management of CVA. Interpretation of FeNO measurement results requires consideration of clinical context, patient symptoms, and other diagnostic findings to confirm the diagnosis of CVA and guide individualized treatment strategies. Incorporating FeNO measurement into the diagnostic algorithm for CVA enhances diagnostic accuracy, facilitates personalized treatment approaches, and improves outcomes for individuals with this distinct clinical phenotype of asthma.

Allergy Testing in the Evaluation of Cough-Variant Asthma

Allergy testing plays a crucial role in the comprehensive evaluation of cough-variant asthma (CVA), aiding in the identification of allergic triggers, allergen sensitization patterns, and potential exacerbating factors contributing to airway inflammation and bronchial hyperresponsiveness. This section explores the principles, methods, interpretation, and clinical significance of allergy testing in the assessment and management of CVA.

1. Principles of Allergy Testing:

Allergy testing aims to identify specific allergens to which an individual is sensitized, triggering an allergic immune response and contributing to the pathogenesis of respiratory conditions such as asthma. The two main types of allergy testing used in the evaluation of CVA are:

- **Skin Prick Testing (SPT):** SPT involves the application of allergen extracts to the skin surface, followed by the introduction of a small puncture or prick to facilitate allergen entry into the epidermis. The skin reaction, characterized by erythema and wheal formation, is measured after a specified period to assess allergen sensitization.
- **Serum Specific IgE Testing:** Serum specific IgE testing, also known as allergy blood testing or allergen-specific IgE testing, measures the concentration of specific IgE antibodies against allergens in the bloodstream. This test provides a quantitative assessment of allergen sensitization and can be performed using various methods, including enzyme-linked immunosorbent assay (ELISA) or radioallergosorbent test (RAST).

2. Methods of Allergy Testing:

Allergy testing is typically performed by trained healthcare professionals in specialized allergy or immunology clinics. The following steps outline the methodology of allergy testing:

- **Patient History:** A detailed medical history is obtained to identify potential allergic triggers, environmental exposures, and symptoms suggestive of allergic disease,

such as allergic rhinitis, atopic dermatitis, or asthma.
- **Allergen Selection:** Based on the patient's clinical history and suspected allergens, a panel of allergens relevant to the individual's geographic region, environmental exposures, and sensitization patterns is selected for testing.
- **Skin Prick Testing:** SPT involves the application of allergen extracts to the skin surface, typically on the forearm or back, followed by the introduction of a small puncture or prick through each allergen extract. The skin reaction is assessed after 15-20 minutes, with positive reactions characterized by erythema and wheal formation.
- **Serum Specific IgE Testing:** Blood samples are collected from the patient, and serum specific IgE levels against specific allergens are measured using commercially available test kits or laboratory assays. Results are reported as quantitative values, typically in kilounits per liter (kU/L), with higher levels indicating greater allergen sensitization.

3. Interpretation of Allergy Testing Results:

Interpretation of allergy testing results requires careful consideration of clinical context, patient symptoms, and other diagnostic findings. Key considerations include:

- **Allergen Sensitization:** Positive allergy test results indicate sensitization to specific allergens, suggesting a potential role in triggering allergic symptoms, exacerbating airway inflammation, and contributing to the pathogenesis of CVA.
- **Relevance to Clinical Symptoms:** Allergy test results should be interpreted in conjunction with the patient's clinical history and symptoms to identify relevant allergens and potential allergic triggers contributing to

cough-variant asthma.
- **Cross-Reactivity:** Cross-reactivity between allergens, particularly among closely related allergen families (e.g., pollen allergens, dust mite allergens), may result in positive allergy test results to multiple allergens, complicating interpretation and management decisions.

4. Clinical Significance of Allergy Testing:

Allergy testing has several clinical applications in the evaluation and management of cough-variant asthma, including:

- **Identifying Allergic Triggers:** Allergy testing helps identify specific allergens triggering allergic symptoms and exacerbating airway inflammation in individuals with CVA, guiding targeted allergen avoidance strategies and environmental control measures.
- **Personalizing Treatment:** Allergy testing results inform personalized treatment approaches, including allergen avoidance measures, pharmacotherapy, and allergen immunotherapy (allergy shots), aimed at reducing allergic symptoms, airway inflammation, and bronchial hyperresponsiveness in individuals with CVA.
- **Monitoring Disease Progression:** Serial allergy testing may be used to monitor changes in allergen sensitization patterns over time, assess disease progression, and guide adjustments to asthma management strategies in individuals with CVA.

Conclusion:

Allergy testing plays a vital role in the comprehensive evaluation and management of cough-variant asthma, aiding in the identification of allergic triggers, allergen sensitization patterns, and potential exacerbating factors contributing to airway inflammation and bronchial hyperresponsiveness. By identifying specific allergens triggering allergic symptoms and exacerbating cough-variant asthma, allergy testing guides targeted allergen avoidance strategies, personalized treatment approaches, and environmental control measures to optimize outcomes for affected individuals. Incorporating allergy testing into the diagnostic algorithm for cough-variant asthma enhances diagnostic accuracy, facilitates personalized treatment decisions, and improves patient care in this distinct clinical phenotype of asthma.

Chest Imaging in Cough-Variant Asthma

Chest imaging plays a critical role in the evaluation of respiratory conditions, including cough-variant asthma (CVA), by providing valuable information about airway anatomy, lung parenchyma, and potential complications. While chest imaging is not typically required for the diagnosis of CVA, it may be indicated in certain clinical scenarios to assess for alternative diagnoses, evaluate for complications, or monitor disease progression. This section explores the principles, indications, modalities, interpretation, and clinical significance of chest imaging in the context of CVA.

1. Principles of Chest Imaging:

Chest imaging encompasses various modalities that provide detailed anatomical and functional information about the thoracic structures, including the lungs, airways, pleura, and mediastinum. The two main modalities used in the evaluation of respiratory conditions are:

- **Chest X-ray (CXR):** CXR is a commonly used imaging modality that provides two-dimensional radiographic images of the chest. It is useful for evaluating lung parenchyma, identifying pulmonary infiltrates, consolidations, atelectasis, pleural effusions, and

mediastinal abnormalities. However, CXR has limited sensitivity for detecting subtle airway abnormalities and may be normal in individuals with CVA.
- **Computed Tomography (CT) Scan:** CT scan is a more sensitive imaging modality that provides detailed cross-sectional images of the chest with higher spatial resolution. It is useful for evaluating airway anatomy, lung parenchyma, bronchial wall thickening, mucous plugging, pulmonary nodules, and other structural abnormalities. High-resolution CT (HRCT) scan is particularly valuable for assessing small airway disease and subtle parenchymal changes associated with asthma.

2. Indications for Chest Imaging in Cough-Variant Asthma:

While chest imaging is not routinely indicated for the diagnosis of CVA, it may be warranted in certain clinical scenarios, including:

- **Atypical Symptoms:** Chest imaging may be indicated in individuals with atypical symptoms, such as hemoptysis, chest pain, or persistent cough refractory to standard asthma therapy, to evaluate for alternative diagnoses, such as pulmonary embolism, pneumonia, bronchiectasis, or malignancy.
- **Complications:** Chest imaging may be indicated in individuals with suspected complications of asthma, such as pneumonia, pneumothorax, pleural effusion, or acute respiratory distress syndrome (ARDS), to assess disease severity, guide management decisions, and monitor response to treatment.
- **Assessment of Disease Severity:** Chest imaging may be indicated in individuals with severe or refractory CVA to assess the extent of airway inflammation, bronchial hyperresponsiveness, and structural changes, such as

airway remodeling, mucous plugging, or parenchymal abnormalities.

3. Interpretation of Chest Imaging Findings:

Interpretation of chest imaging findings requires careful consideration of clinical context, patient symptoms, and other diagnostic findings. Key considerations include:

- **Airway Abnormalities:** Chest imaging may reveal bronchial wall thickening, mucous plugging, bronchiectasis, or air trapping suggestive of airway inflammation and remodeling in individuals with CVA.
- **Parenchymal Changes:** Chest imaging may show peribronchial cuffing, ground-glass opacities, or areas of consolidation suggestive of airway inflammation, atelectasis, or infection in individuals with CVA.
- **Complications:** Chest imaging may identify complications of asthma, such as pneumonia, pneumothorax, pleural effusion, or pulmonary embolism, which may require specific management strategies and interventions.

4. Clinical Significance of Chest Imaging:

Chest imaging has several clinical applications in the evaluation and management of CVA, including:

- **Diagnostic Evaluation:** Chest imaging helps rule out alternative diagnoses, assess disease severity, and guide management decisions in individuals with CVA presenting with atypical symptoms or complications.
- **Treatment Monitoring:** Serial chest imaging may be used to monitor disease progression, assess treatment response, and guide adjustments to asthma management strategies in individuals with severe or refractory CVA.
- **Complication Detection:** Chest imaging helps identify

complications of asthma, such as pneumonia, pneumothorax, or pulmonary embolism, which may require prompt recognition and targeted interventions to optimize outcomes.

Conclusion:

Chest imaging plays a valuable role in the evaluation and management of cough-variant asthma, providing important diagnostic information about airway anatomy, lung parenchyma, and potential complications. While chest imaging is not routinely indicated for the diagnosis of CVA, it may be warranted in certain clinical scenarios to assess for alternative diagnoses, evaluate disease severity, or monitor treatment response. Interpretation of chest imaging findings requires careful consideration of clinical context, patient symptoms, and other diagnostic findings to guide individualized management strategies and optimize outcomes for individuals with CVA. Incorporating chest imaging into the diagnostic algorithm for CVA enhances diagnostic accuracy, facilitates prompt recognition of complications, and improves patient care in this distinct clinical phenotype of asthma.

Differential Diagnosis of Cough-Variant Asthma

Cough is a common symptom encountered in clinical practice and can be attributed to a wide range of etiologies, including respiratory, cardiac, gastrointestinal, neurological, and systemic conditions. Cough-variant asthma (CVA) represents a distinct clinical phenotype of asthma characterized by isolated cough as the predominant symptom in the absence of typical wheezing or dyspnea. However, the diagnosis of CVA can be challenging due to its overlapping clinical features with other conditions. This section explores the differential diagnosis of cough-variant asthma, highlighting key differential diagnostic considerations, evaluation strategies, and distinguishing features of various conditions.

1. Asthma Phenotypes:

- **Classic Asthma:** Classic asthma presents with the triad of cough, wheezing, and dyspnea, with variable degrees of airflow obstruction and airway hyperresponsiveness. Unlike CVA, classic asthma typically involves wheezing and may present with other symptoms such as chest tightness and shortness of breath.
- **Allergic Asthma:** Allergic asthma is characterized by airway inflammation and hyperresponsiveness triggered by allergen exposure, leading to cough, wheezing, and dyspnea. Individuals with allergic asthma may have a history of allergic rhinitis, eczema, or other atopic conditions, which can help differentiate it from CVA.

2. Upper Airway Conditions:

- **Postnasal Drip:** Postnasal drip syndrome is characterized by the sensation of mucus dripping down the back of the throat, leading to throat irritation and cough. It is commonly caused by allergic rhinitis, sinusitis, or upper respiratory tract infections and may present with nasal congestion, throat clearing, and cough, mimicking symptoms of CVA.
- **Chronic Rhinosinusitis:** Chronic rhinosinusitis is characterized by inflammation of the nasal and sinus mucosa, leading to nasal congestion, postnasal drip, facial pain, and cough. Individuals with chronic rhinosinusitis may have purulent nasal discharge, facial pressure, and anosmia, which can help differentiate it from CVA.

3. Gastroesophageal Conditions:

- **Gastroesophageal Reflux Disease (GERD):** GERD is characterized by the reflux of gastric contents into the esophagus, leading to heartburn, regurgitation, and cough. Acid reflux-induced cough may occur predominantly at night or upon lying down and may be associated with a sour taste in the mouth, throat irritation, and hoarseness.
- **Laryngopharyngeal Reflux (LPR):** LPR is a variant of GERD characterized by reflux of gastric contents into the larynx and pharynx, leading to throat clearing, hoarseness, and chronic cough. LPR-related cough may be exacerbated by eating, drinking, or lying down and may be accompanied by globus sensation or throat discomfort.

4. **Respiratory Infections:**

   - **Acute Bronchitis:** Acute bronchitis is characterized by inflammation of the bronchial mucosa, typically following viral respiratory infections, leading to cough, sputum production, and chest discomfort. Unlike CVA, acute bronchitis is often associated with systemic symptoms such as fever, malaise, and myalgias and may resolve spontaneously within 1-3 weeks.
   - **Pneumonia:** Pneumonia is characterized by inflammation of the lung parenchyma, typically due to bacterial, viral, or atypical pathogens, leading to cough, fever, dyspnea, and pleuritic chest pain. Unlike CVA, pneumonia may present with focal lung findings such as consolidation, crackles, and dullness to percussion on physical examination.

5. **Cardiac Conditions:**

   - **Congestive Heart Failure (CHF):** CHF is characterized by impaired cardiac function leading to fluid overload, pulmonary congestion, and cough. CHF-related cough is typically paroxysmal, worse at night, and may be accompanied by dyspnea on exertion, orthopnea, and peripheral edema. Unlike CVA, CHF-related cough is often associated with signs of volume overload on physical examination, such as crackles and elevated jugular venous pressure.

- **Left Ventricular Dysfunction:** Left ventricular dysfunction can lead to pulmonary congestion and interstitial edema, resulting in cough and dyspnea. Individuals with left ventricular dysfunction may have a history of coronary artery disease, hypertension, or valvular heart disease, which can help differentiate it from CVA.

6. Miscellaneous Conditions:

- **Medication-Induced Cough:** Certain medications, such as angiotensin-converting enzyme (ACE) inhibitors, beta-blockers, and angiotensin receptor blockers (ARBs), can cause cough as a side effect. Medication-induced cough typically occurs shortly after initiating therapy and may resolve upon discontinuation of the offending agent.
- **Psychogenic Cough:** Psychogenic cough, also known as habit cough or tic cough, is characterized by repetitive coughing in the absence of underlying respiratory or organic pathology. Psychogenic cough may be triggered by stress, anxiety, or psychological factors and typically persists despite medical treatment.

Conclusion:

The differential diagnosis of cough-variant asthma encompasses a wide range of conditions, including other asthma phenotypes, upper airway conditions, gastroesophageal disorders, respiratory infections, cardiac conditions, medication-induced cough, and psychogenic cough. Distinguishing cough-variant asthma from other etiologies requires a thorough clinical evaluation, including detailed history-taking, physical examination, diagnostic testing, and consideration of clinical context. By systematically considering differential diagnostic considerations and evaluating for specific features suggestive of alternative diagnoses, healthcare providers can accurately diagnose cough-variant asthma and initiate appropriate management strategies to optimize outcomes for affected individuals.

CHAPTER 5: MANAGEMENT AND TREATMENT STRATEGIES

Pharmacological Interventions in Cough-Variant Asthma

Cough-variant asthma (CVA) is a distinct clinical phenotype of asthma characterized by isolated cough as the predominant symptom. While the underlying pathophysiology of CVA shares similarities with classic asthma, management strategies may differ due to the absence of typical wheezing or dyspnea. Pharmacological interventions play a central role in the treatment of CVA, aiming to reduce airway inflammation, bronchial hyperresponsiveness, and cough frequency. This section explores the pharmacological agents commonly used in the management of CVA, including inhaled corticosteroids, beta2-agonists, leukotriene modifiers, mast cell stabilizers, anti-IgE therapy, oral corticosteroids, and immunomodulators.

Pharmacological Interventions:

Inhaled Corticosteroids:

Inhaled corticosteroids (ICS) are the cornerstone of asthma therapy and serve as first-line treatment for CVA. These medications exert potent anti-inflammatory effects on the airways, reducing airway inflammation, mucosal edema, and bronchial hyperresponsiveness. Commonly used ICS agents include:

- **Beclomethasone (Qvar)**
- **Budesonide (Pulmicort)**
- **Fluticasone (Flovent)**
- **Mometasone (Asmanex)**

ICS are typically administered via metered-dose inhalers (MDIs) or dry powder inhalers (DPIs) to ensure targeted delivery to the lungs. Regular use of ICS has been shown to improve cough frequency, lung function, and quality of life in individuals with CVA.

Beta2-Agonists:

Beta2-agonists are bronchodilators that act on beta2-adrenergic receptors in the airway smooth muscle, leading to relaxation of bronchial smooth muscle and relief of bronchospasm. Short-acting beta2-agonists (SABAs) provide rapid symptomatic relief of cough and bronchospasm, while long-acting beta2-agonists (LABAs) offer sustained bronchodilation and are used for maintenance therapy. Commonly used beta2-agonists include:

- **Short-Acting Beta2-Agonists (SABAs):**
    - Albuterol (Ventolin, Proventil)
    - Levalbuterol (Xopenex)
- **Long-Acting Beta2-Agonists (LABAs):**
    - Salmeterol (Serevent)
    - Formoterol (Foradil)

Beta2-agonists are typically administered via MDIs or nebulizers and may be used as rescue medication for acute symptom relief or as adjunctive therapy for persistent symptoms in individuals with CVA.

Leukotriene Modifiers:

Leukotriene modifiers are oral medications that inhibit the action of leukotrienes, potent inflammatory mediators involved in the pathogenesis of asthma. These medications exert anti-inflammatory effects, reducing airway inflammation, bronchial hyperresponsiveness, and mucus production. Commonly used leukotriene modifiers include:

- **Montelukast (Singulair)**
- **Zafirlukast (Accolate)**
- **Zileuton (Zyflo)**

Leukotriene modifiers are typically used as adjunctive therapy in individuals with CVA who remain symptomatic despite treatment with ICS or beta2-agonists. These medications are particularly beneficial in individuals with concomitant allergic rhinitis or aspirin-exacerbated respiratory disease.

Mast Cell Stabilizers:

Mast cell stabilizers are medications that inhibit the release of inflammatory mediators from mast cells, including histamine, leukotrienes, and cytokines. These medications exert anti-inflammatory and bronchodilator effects, reducing airway inflammation and bronchial hyperresponsiveness. Commonly used mast cell stabilizers include:

- **Cromolyn sodium (Intal)**
- **Nedocromil (Tilade)**

Mast cell stabilizers are typically administered via inhalation and may be used as adjunctive therapy in individuals with CVA who have exercise-induced symptoms or who are unable to tolerate other asthma medications.

Anti-IgE Therapy:

Anti-IgE therapy targets immunoglobulin E (IgE), a key mediator of allergic inflammation in asthma. This biologic therapy binds to circulating IgE antibodies, preventing their interaction with mast cells and basophils and inhibiting the release of inflammatory mediators. Omalizumab (Xolair) is the only anti-IgE therapy currently approved for the treatment of asthma. It is administered via subcutaneous injection every 2-4 weeks and is indicated for individuals with severe allergic asthma who have persistent symptoms despite treatment with ICS and other controller medications.

Oral Corticosteroids:

Oral corticosteroids (OCS) are potent anti-inflammatory medications that are used for short-term management of acute exacerbations or severe persistent symptoms in individuals with CVA. These medications exert broad-spectrum anti-inflammatory effects, reducing airway inflammation, mucosal edema, and bronchial hyperresponsiveness. Commonly used OCS include:

- **Prednisone**
- **Prednisolone**
- **Methylprednisolone**
- **Dexamethasone**

OCS are typically reserved for short-term use due to their potential for adverse effects, including systemic immunosuppression, osteoporosis, glucose intolerance, and adrenal suppression. Long-term use of OCS should be avoided whenever possible, and alternative maintenance therapies should be considered for individuals with persistent symptoms.

Immunomodulators:

Immunomodulators are a diverse group of medications that modulate immune responses and inflammatory pathways involved in the pathogenesis of asthma. These medications exert anti-inflammatory effects, reducing airway inflammation, bronchial hyperresponsiveness, and mucus production. Commonly used immunomodulators include:

- **Methotrexate**
- **Cyclosporine**
- **Tacrolimus**
- **Azathioprine**

Immunomodulators are typically reserved for individuals with severe or refractory CVA who have failed to respond to conventional asthma therapies. These medications may be used as adjunctive therapy in combination with ICS, beta2-agonists, or other controller medications to achieve optimal asthma control.

Conclusion:

Pharmacological interventions play a central role in the management of cough-variant asthma, aiming to reduce airway inflammation, bronchial hyperresponsiveness, and cough frequency. Inhaled corticosteroids, beta2-agonists, leukotriene modifiers, mast cell stabilizers, anti-IgE therapy, oral corticosteroids, and immunomodulators are among the pharmacological agents commonly used in the treatment of CVA. By targeting underlying inflammatory pathways and bronchial hyperreactivity, these medications help alleviate symptoms, improve lung function, and enhance quality of life in individuals with CVA. Dosing, administration, and monitoring of pharmacological therapies should be individualized based on disease severity, treatment response, and potential adverse effects to optimize outcomes for affected individuals. Close collaboration between healthcare providers and patients is essential to develop personalized treatment plans and achieve optimal asthma control in this distinct clinical phenotype of asthma.

Non-Pharmacological Approaches in the Management of Cough-Variant Asthma

Cough-variant asthma (CVA) represents a unique clinical phenotype of asthma characterized by isolated cough as the predominant symptom. While pharmacological interventions play a central role in controlling airway inflammation and bronchial hyperresponsiveness, non-pharmacological approaches are also integral components of comprehensive asthma management. These approaches aim to reduce cough frequency, improve lung function, and enhance quality of life through trigger avoidance, respiratory therapy and education, lifestyle modifications, and psychological support. This section explores the importance, principles, and practical implementation of non-pharmacological interventions in the management of CVA.

Non-Pharmacological Approaches:

Trigger Avoidance:

Identifying and avoiding triggers that exacerbate cough and airway inflammation is fundamental to the management of CVA. Common triggers may include allergens, irritants, respiratory infections, exercise, changes in weather, and occupational exposures. Trigger avoidance strategies may include:

- **Allergen Avoidance:** Individuals with allergic asthma should minimize exposure to environmental allergens such as pollen, dust mites, pet dander, and mold. This may involve using allergen-proof bedding, air purifiers, and avoiding outdoor activities during high pollen seasons.

- **Irritant Avoidance:** Minimizing exposure to respiratory irritants such as tobacco smoke, air pollution, strong odors, and chemical fumes is essential in reducing cough frequency and airway inflammation. This may involve implementing smoke-free policies at home and work, using air filtration systems, and avoiding harsh cleaning products.
- **Respiratory Infection Prevention:** Practicing good hand hygiene, avoiding close contact with individuals who are sick, and receiving recommended vaccinations (e.g., influenza, pneumococcal) can help reduce the risk of respiratory infections, which can exacerbate cough and asthma symptoms.
- **Exercise Modification:** Individuals with exercise-induced cough may benefit from pre-exercise bronchodilator therapy, warm-up exercises, and avoiding cold or dry environments. Engaging in low-impact activities such as swimming or cycling may also be beneficial for individuals with exercise-induced symptoms.

Respiratory Therapy and Education:

Respiratory therapy and education are essential components of asthma management, providing individuals with CVA with the knowledge and skills necessary to optimize their respiratory health and achieve optimal asthma control. Key components of respiratory therapy and education include:

- **Asthma Action Plan:** Developing a personalized asthma action plan in collaboration with healthcare providers empowers individuals with CVA to recognize worsening symptoms, initiate appropriate self-management strategies, and seek timely medical intervention when needed. Asthma action plans typically include instructions for medication use, symptom monitoring, and steps to take in case of worsening symptoms or asthma exacerbations.

- **Inhaler Technique Training:** Proper inhaler technique is essential for the effective delivery of medication to the lungs and optimal asthma control. Healthcare providers should educate individuals with CVA on correct inhaler technique, including proper device priming, breath coordination, and mouthpiece or mask seal.
- **Peak Flow Monitoring:** Peak flow monitoring allows individuals with CVA to assess their lung function and monitor for changes in airflow obstruction. Regular peak flow measurements, recorded in an asthma diary or smartphone application, provide valuable information about asthma control and treatment response.
- **Triggers Identification:** Educating individuals with CVA about common asthma triggers, including allergens, irritants, respiratory infections, and exercise, helps them recognize and avoid potential exacerbating factors. Healthcare providers should provide guidance on trigger avoidance strategies and environmental control measures to minimize exposure to known triggers.

Lifestyle Modifications:

Adopting healthy lifestyle habits can help individuals with CVA optimize their respiratory health, reduce cough frequency, and improve overall well-being. Lifestyle modifications may include:

- **Smoking Cessation:** Smoking is a major risk factor for asthma development and exacerbations and can worsen cough and airway inflammation. Individuals with CVA who smoke should be encouraged to quit smoking and provided with smoking cessation support resources.

- **Healthy Diet:** A balanced diet rich in fruits, vegetables, whole grains, and lean proteins can support immune function, reduce inflammation, and improve respiratory health. Healthcare providers should provide nutrition education and guidance on healthy eating habits for individuals with CVA.
- **Regular Exercise:** Regular physical activity is important for maintaining cardiovascular health, improving lung function, and reducing asthma symptoms. Individuals with CVA should be encouraged to engage in regular exercise, tailored to their fitness level and preferences, to enhance respiratory fitness and overall well-being.
- **Stress Management:** Psychological stress can exacerbate asthma symptoms and increase cough frequency. Stress management techniques such as deep breathing exercises, meditation, yoga, and relaxation techniques can help individuals with CVA reduce stress levels and improve asthma control.

Psychological Support:

Living with a chronic respiratory condition such as CVA can be challenging and may impact emotional well-being and quality of life. Psychological support and counseling can help individuals with CVA cope with the challenges of asthma and develop effective coping strategies. Key components of psychological support may include:

- **Cognitive-Behavioral Therapy (CBT):** CBT is a structured, evidence-based psychotherapy approach that helps individuals with CVA identify and modify maladaptive thoughts and behaviors related to asthma management. CBT techniques such as relaxation training, stress management, and cognitive restructuring can help individuals develop coping skills and improve asthma self-management.

- **Support Groups:** Participating in asthma support groups or online forums allows individuals with CVA to connect with others who share similar experiences, exchange information, and provide mutual support. Support groups provide a sense of community, validation, and empowerment for individuals living with asthma.
- **Psychiatric Evaluation:** Individuals with CVA experiencing significant psychological distress, anxiety, or depression may benefit from psychiatric evaluation and treatment. Psychiatric medications, such as selective serotonin reuptake inhibitors (SSRIs) or serotonin-norepinephrine reuptake inhibitors (SNRIs), may be prescribed to manage mood symptoms and improve overall well-being.

Conclusion:

Non-pharmacological approaches play a vital role in the comprehensive management of cough-variant asthma, complementing pharmacological interventions to optimize respiratory health and improve quality of life. Trigger avoidance strategies, respiratory therapy and education, lifestyle modifications, and psychological support are integral components of asthma management, empowering individuals with CVA to effectively manage their condition, reduce cough frequency, and achieve optimal asthma control. By addressing modifiable risk factors, promoting healthy lifestyle habits, and providing psychological support, healthcare providers can help individuals with CVA enhance their respiratory health and overall well-being, leading to improved asthma outcomes and enhanced quality of life.

Acute Management of Exacerbations in Cough-Variant Asthma

Acute exacerbations of cough-variant asthma (CVA) represent significant clinical challenges requiring prompt recognition and intervention to prevent respiratory compromise and optimize outcomes. While individuals with CVA may not present with typical wheezing or dyspnea, exacerbations can manifest as worsening cough, respiratory distress, and impaired lung function. This section delves into the acute management of CVA exacerbations, focusing on bronchodilators, systemic corticosteroids, oxygen therapy, and intensive care management.

Acute Management of Exacerbations:

Bronchodilators:

Bronchodilators are central to the acute management of CVA exacerbations, providing rapid relief of bronchospasm and improving airflow obstruction. Short-acting beta2-agonists (SABAs) such as albuterol are the mainstay of bronchodilator therapy and are typically administered via metered-dose inhalers (MDIs) or nebulizers. The administration of SABAs results in smooth muscle relaxation, leading to bronchodilation and alleviation of respiratory symptoms. In acute exacerbations, SABAs may be administered at higher doses and more frequent intervals to achieve rapid symptom relief. Inhaled anticholinergic agents such as ipratropium bromide may be used as adjunctive therapy in individuals with severe exacerbations or inadequate response to SABAs.

Systemic Corticosteroids:

Systemic corticosteroids play a crucial role in the acute management of CVA exacerbations by reducing airway inflammation and improving lung function. Oral corticosteroids (OCS) such as prednisone or prednisolone are typically initiated early in the management of exacerbations and continued for a short course (e.g., 3-7 days) to hasten symptom resolution and prevent relapse. OCS exert broad anti-inflammatory effects, including suppression of cytokine production, inhibition of inflammatory cell migration, and reduction of airway edema. In individuals with severe exacerbations or those unable to tolerate oral medications, intravenous corticosteroids may be administered in a hospital setting.

Oxygen Therapy:

Oxygen therapy is essential in the management of CVA exacerbations, particularly in individuals with severe respiratory distress or hypoxemia. Supplemental oxygen should be titrated to achieve target oxygen saturations (> 90%) and alleviate hypoxemia while avoiding hyperoxia and potential oxygen toxicity. Oxygen delivery systems may include nasal cannula, face mask, or high-flow nasal cannula depending on the severity of respiratory compromise and patient tolerance. Continuous monitoring of oxygen saturation, respiratory rate, and clinical status is essential to guide oxygen therapy titration and ensure adequate tissue oxygenation.

Intensive Care Management:

In severe or life-threatening CVA exacerbations, intensive care management may be required to provide advanced respiratory support, hemodynamic stabilization, and close monitoring of clinical status. Individuals with severe exacerbations may present with respiratory failure, altered mental status, hemodynamic instability, or signs of impending respiratory arrest. Intensive care management strategies may include:

- **Mechanical Ventilation:** Invasive or non-invasive mechanical ventilation may be necessary in individuals with severe respiratory distress, impending respiratory failure, or inadequate response to conventional therapies. Mechanical ventilation aims to provide

adequate oxygenation and ventilation while minimizing respiratory effort and work of breathing.
- **Continuous Monitoring:** Close monitoring of vital signs, oxygen saturation, respiratory mechanics, and laboratory parameters is essential to assess response to treatment, detect complications, and guide therapeutic interventions. Continuous cardiac monitoring and invasive hemodynamic monitoring may be indicated in individuals with hemodynamic instability or shock.
- **Bronchodilator Therapy:** Continuous or frequent administration of bronchodilators may be required in individuals with severe exacerbations to achieve bronchodilation and alleviate airway obstruction. Continuous nebulization or administration of bronchodilators via metered-dose inhalers with spacers may be used to maintain airway patency and improve gas exchange.
- **Systemic Corticosteroids:** Intravenous corticosteroids may be administered in individuals with severe exacerbations or those unable to tolerate oral medications to rapidly suppress airway inflammation and reduce the risk of treatment failure or relapse.
- **Adjunctive Therapies:** Adjunctive therapies such as magnesium sulfate, heliox, or intravenous bronchodilators (e.g., terbutaline) may be considered in refractory cases or as rescue therapy in individuals with severe exacerbations unresponsive to conventional treatments.

Conclusion:

Acute exacerbations of cough-variant asthma require prompt recognition, aggressive intervention, and close monitoring to prevent respiratory compromise and optimize outcomes. Bronchodilators, systemic corticosteroids, oxygen therapy, and intensive care management are integral components of the acute management of CVA exacerbations, aiming to alleviate symptoms, improve lung function, and prevent progression to respiratory failure. Timely administration of bronchodilators and systemic corticosteroids is essential to reduce airway inflammation, relieve bronchospasm, and hasten symptom resolution. Oxygen therapy should be titrated to achieve target oxygen saturations while avoiding hyperoxia and potential oxygen toxicity. In severe or life-threatening exacerbations, intensive care management may be required to provide advanced respiratory support, hemodynamic stabilization, and continuous monitoring of clinical status. By implementing evidence-based management strategies and individualizing treatment approaches based on disease severity and patient response, healthcare providers can optimize outcomes and improve prognosis in individuals experiencing acute exacerbations of cough-variant asthma.

Long-Term Monitoring and Follow-Up in Cough-Variant Asthma

Cough-variant asthma (CVA) requires long-term monitoring and follow-up to ensure optimal disease control, prevent exacerbations, and address evolving clinical needs. Unlike classic asthma, which may present with wheezing or dyspnea, CVA is characterized primarily by cough as the predominant symptom. However, despite the absence of typical symptoms, individuals with CVA are still at risk of experiencing asthma exacerbations and long-term complications. This section explores the importance of long-term monitoring and follow-up in CVA, focusing on assessment strategies, treatment adjustments, patient education, and lifestyle modifications.

Importance of Long-Term Monitoring and Follow-Up:

Long-term monitoring and follow-up play a crucial role in the management of CVA, allowing healthcare providers to assess disease control, monitor treatment response, and address potential complications. Regular follow-up visits provide opportunities for healthcare providers to evaluate symptoms, lung function, medication adherence, and asthma triggers, and adjust treatment plans accordingly. Additionally, long-term monitoring helps identify emerging comorbidities, such as allergic rhinitis, gastroesophageal reflux disease (GERD), or sleep-disordered breathing, which may impact asthma control and require targeted management strategies.

Assessment Strategies:

During long-term monitoring and follow-up visits, healthcare providers utilize various assessment strategies to evaluate disease control and treatment response in individuals with CVA. Key components of the assessment may include:

- **Symptom Evaluation:** Assessing the frequency, severity, and impact of cough on daily activities helps gauge disease control and treatment effectiveness. Individuals with well-controlled CVA may experience minimal coughing episodes, while those with poorly controlled asthma may report persistent or worsening symptoms despite treatment.
- **Lung Function Testing:** Performing spirometry or peak expiratory flow (PEF) monitoring provides objective measures of airflow obstruction and helps assess lung function over time. Changes in spirometry parameters, such as forced expiratory volume in one second (FEV1) or forced vital capacity (FVC), may indicate worsening asthma control or treatment response.
- **Asthma Control Questionnaires:** Utilizing standardized asthma control questionnaires, such as the Asthma Control Test (ACT) or the Childhood Asthma Control Test

(C-ACT), helps assess overall asthma control and guide treatment decisions. These questionnaires evaluate symptoms, medication use, and functional impairment and provide a quantitative measure of asthma control.

- **Medication Adherence:** Reviewing medication adherence and inhaler technique ensures that individuals with CVA are using their medications correctly and consistently. Poor medication adherence or incorrect inhaler technique may contribute to inadequate asthma control and exacerbations and require targeted education and intervention.
- **Identification of Triggers:** Identifying and addressing asthma triggers, such as allergens, irritants, respiratory infections, or exercise, helps minimize exposure and reduce the risk of exacerbations. Healthcare providers should inquire about potential triggers during follow-up visits and provide guidance on trigger avoidance strategies and environmental control measures.

Treatment Adjustments:

Based on the assessment findings during long-term monitoring and follow-up, healthcare providers may adjust treatment plans to optimize asthma control and reduce the risk of exacerbations. Treatment adjustments may include:

- **Medication Optimization:** Up-titration of controller medications, such as inhaled corticosteroids (ICS) or leukotriene modifiers, may be necessary to achieve adequate asthma control in individuals with persistent symptoms or exacerbations. Addition of long-acting beta2-agonists (LABAs) or anti-IgE therapy may be considered in individuals with uncontrolled CVA despite optimized ICS therapy.
- **Stepwise Approach:** Following a stepwise approach to asthma management, as outlined in national

and international guidelines (e.g., Global Initiative for Asthma [GINA]), helps guide treatment decisions based on disease severity and control. Healthcare providers should periodically reassess asthma control and adjust treatment regimens accordingly, moving up or down the treatment ladder as needed to achieve optimal outcomes.
- **Comorbidity Management:** Addressing comorbid conditions that may impact asthma control, such as allergic rhinitis, GERD, or obstructive sleep apnea, is essential in individuals with CVA. Targeted management of comorbidities may improve asthma control, reduce exacerbations, and enhance overall quality of life.

Patient Education and Empowerment:

Long-term monitoring and follow-up visits provide opportunities for patient education and empowerment, enabling individuals with CVA to actively participate in their asthma management and make informed decisions about their health. Key components of patient education may include:

- **Asthma Self-Management:** Educating individuals with CVA about asthma self-management techniques, including proper inhaler technique, medication adherence, trigger avoidance, and asthma action plans, empowers them to take control of their asthma and respond effectively to worsening symptoms or exacerbations.
- **Lifestyle Modifications:** Providing guidance on lifestyle modifications, such as smoking cessation, healthy diet, regular exercise, stress management, and environmental control measures, helps individuals with CVA optimize their respiratory health and reduce the risk of exacerbations.
- **Recognizing Warning Signs:** Educating individuals with CVA about the warning signs of worsening asthma, such

as increasing cough frequency, shortness of breath, chest tightness, or nocturnal symptoms, helps them recognize early signs of exacerbations and seek timely medical intervention.
- **Follow-Up Planning:** Scheduling regular follow-up visits and establishing open communication channels between healthcare providers and individuals with CVA ensure ongoing monitoring, support, and adjustment of treatment plans as needed. Telehealth or virtual visits may be utilized to facilitate access to care and enhance patient engagement, particularly in individuals with limited mobility or transportation barriers.

Conclusion:

Long-term monitoring and follow-up are essential components of the comprehensive management of cough-variant asthma, allowing healthcare providers to assess disease control, monitor treatment response, and address evolving clinical needs. Assessment strategies, treatment adjustments, patient education, and empowerment are integral components of long-term asthma management, enabling individuals with CVA to achieve optimal asthma control, prevent exacerbations, and enhance overall quality of life. By implementing evidence-based monitoring protocols, individualized treatment plans, and patient-centered education strategies, healthcare providers can optimize outcomes and improve prognosis in individuals living with CVA.

CHAPTER 6: COMPLICATIONS AND COMORBIDITIES

Chronic Obstructive Pulmonary Disease (COPD) in the Context of Cough-Variant Asthma

Chronic Obstructive Pulmonary Disease (COPD) represents a significant respiratory condition characterized by persistent airflow limitation and respiratory symptoms, typically including chronic cough, sputum production, and dyspnea. While COPD and cough-variant asthma (CVA) are distinct respiratory conditions, they share overlapping clinical features and may present diagnostic and management challenges. This section explores the relationship between COPD and CVA, highlighting key similarities, differences, and implications for diagnosis and management.

Understanding COPD:

COPD encompasses a group of progressive lung diseases, including chronic bronchitis and emphysema, characterized by airflow limitation and irreversible damage to the airways and lung parenchyma. The primary risk factor for COPD development is tobacco smoking, although exposure to environmental pollutants, occupational dusts and chemicals, and genetic predisposition may also contribute to disease pathogenesis. COPD is associated with chronic inflammation, mucus hypersecretion, airway remodeling, and alveolar destruction, leading to airflow obstruction, gas trapping, and impaired gas exchange.

Clinical Features of COPD:

The hallmark symptoms of COPD include chronic cough, sputum production, and dyspnea, which typically worsen over time and significantly impact quality of life. Individuals with COPD may experience exacerbations characterized by acute worsening of respiratory symptoms, often triggered by respiratory infections, environmental pollutants, or other factors. Physical examination findings in COPD may include wheezing, decreased breath sounds, hyperinflation of the chest, and signs of respiratory distress.

Diagnosis of COPD:

The diagnosis of COPD is based on a combination of clinical history, physical examination, and objective testing, including spirometry. Spirometry demonstrates airflow limitation characterized by a reduced ratio of forced expiratory volume in one second (FEV1) to forced vital capacity (FVC) after bronchodilator administration. Additional tests, such as chest imaging (e.g., chest X-ray or computed tomography [CT] scan) and arterial blood gas analysis, may be performed to assess disease severity and evaluate for complications such as pulmonary hypertension or cor pulmonale.

Treatment of COPD:

The management of COPD aims to reduce symptoms, prevent disease progression, improve quality of life, and reduce the risk of exacerbations. Key components of COPD management include smoking cessation, pharmacological therapy, pulmonary rehabilitation, oxygen therapy, and vaccination against respiratory infections. Bronchodilators, including short-acting and long-acting beta2-agonists and anticholinergic agents, are central to symptom management and bronchodilation in COPD. Inhaled corticosteroids may be used in combination with bronchodilators for individuals with frequent exacerbations or severe airflow limitation.

Understanding the Relationship between COPD and CVA:

While COPD and CVA are distinct respiratory conditions, they share overlapping clinical features, including chronic cough and airflow limitation. In some cases, individuals with COPD may present with cough as the predominant symptom, resembling the clinical phenotype of CVA. Additionally, individuals with CVA may develop fixed airflow limitation and airway remodeling over time, resembling features of COPD. The presence of overlapping symptoms and pathophysiological mechanisms can complicate the diagnosis and management of these conditions, necessitating a comprehensive evaluation and individualized treatment approach.

Implications for Diagnosis and Management:

The diagnosis and management of individuals with overlapping features of COPD and CVA require careful consideration of clinical history, symptomatology, objective testing, and treatment response. Differential diagnosis may be challenging, particularly in individuals with a history of smoking or occupational exposures. Spirometry remains essential in distinguishing between COPD and CVA, as airflow limitation is a hallmark feature of COPD but may be absent or reversible in CVA. Comorbidities, such as allergic rhinitis, GERD, or cardiovascular disease, may further complicate the clinical picture and require targeted evaluation and management.

Conclusion:

COPD and CVA represent distinct respiratory conditions characterized by airflow limitation and chronic cough, respectively. However, overlapping clinical features and pathophysiological mechanisms may complicate the diagnosis and management of individuals with COPD and CVA. A comprehensive evaluation, including clinical history, physical examination, and objective testing, is essential to differentiate between these conditions and develop individualized treatment plans. By understanding the relationship between COPD and CVA and addressing overlapping symptoms and comorbidities, healthcare providers can optimize outcomes and improve quality of life for individuals living with these chronic respiratory conditions.

Bronchiectasis: Understanding a Chronic Respiratory Condition

Bronchiectasis is a chronic respiratory condition characterized by irreversible dilatation and thickening of the bronchial walls, leading to impaired mucociliary clearance, recurrent respiratory infections, and persistent cough with sputum production. While bronchiectasis shares clinical features such as chronic cough with conditions like cough-variant asthma (CVA), it presents distinct pathophysiological mechanisms and diagnostic challenges. This section explores bronchiectasis in depth, including its etiology, clinical presentation, diagnosis, management, and its relationship with other respiratory conditions.

Understanding Bronchiectasis:

Bronchiectasis results from the destruction and widening of the airway walls, which impairs the ability of the airways to clear mucus effectively. This leads to mucus retention, chronic inflammation, and recurrent respiratory infections. While bronchiectasis may develop secondary to conditions such as cystic fibrosis, primary ciliary dyskinesia, or immunodeficiency disorders, it can also occur idiopathically or as a consequence of previous respiratory infections or inhalation of irritants.

Clinical Presentation of Bronchiectasis:

The clinical presentation of bronchiectasis varies widely but commonly includes symptoms such as chronic cough, often with purulent sputum production, recurrent respiratory infections, dyspnea, and fatigue. Individuals with bronchiectasis may experience exacerbations characterized by worsening respiratory symptoms, increased sputum production, and acute respiratory distress. Physical examination findings may include crackles, wheezing, and clubbing of the fingers, particularly in advanced disease.

Diagnosis of Bronchiectasis:

The diagnosis of bronchiectasis requires a combination of clinical evaluation, radiological imaging, and pulmonary function testing. High-resolution computed tomography (HRCT) of the chest is the gold standard for diagnosing bronchiectasis, demonstrating characteristic findings such as bronchial dilatation, bronchial wall thickening, and mucous plugging. Pulmonary function tests may reveal airflow obstruction, reduced lung volumes, and impaired gas exchange in advanced disease.

Management of Bronchiectasis:

The management of bronchiectasis aims to reduce symptoms, prevent exacerbations, and improve quality of life through a combination of pharmacological and non-pharmacological interventions. Key components of bronchiectasis management include:

- **Airway Clearance Techniques:** Regular airway clearance techniques, such as chest physiotherapy, postural drainage, percussion, and vibration, help mobilize and remove excess mucus from the airways, reducing the risk of infection and improving lung function.
- **Pharmacological Therapy:** Pharmacological therapy for bronchiectasis may include antibiotics to treat respiratory infections, bronchodilators to alleviate airflow obstruction, and mucolytic agents to reduce sputum viscosity and enhance mucus clearance.
- **Immunization:** Vaccination against respiratory pathogens, including influenza and pneumococcal vaccines, is essential in individuals with bronchiectasis to reduce the risk of respiratory infections and prevent exacerbations.
- **Smoking Cessation:** Smoking cessation is paramount in individuals with bronchiectasis, as smoking exacerbates airway inflammation, impairs mucociliary clearance, and increases the risk of respiratory infections and disease progression.
- **Pulmonary Rehabilitation:** Pulmonary rehabilitation programs, including exercise training, education, and psychosocial support, help improve exercise tolerance, reduce dyspnea, and enhance quality of life in individuals with bronchiectasis.

Relationship with Other Respiratory Conditions:

Bronchiectasis shares overlapping clinical features and risk factors with other respiratory conditions, including COPD, asthma, and cystic fibrosis. Individuals with bronchiectasis may also develop comorbidities such as GERD, obstructive sleep apnea, and allergic rhinitis, which can impact disease severity and treatment outcomes. The presence of bronchiectasis in individuals with asthma or COPD may complicate disease management and require targeted evaluation and treatment of bronchial dilatation and mucus clearance impairment.

Conclusion:

Bronchiectasis is a chronic respiratory condition characterized by irreversible dilatation of the bronchial walls, impaired mucociliary clearance, and recurrent respiratory infections. While bronchiectasis shares clinical features such as chronic cough with other respiratory conditions like cough-variant asthma, it presents distinct pathophysiological mechanisms and diagnostic challenges. A comprehensive approach to the diagnosis and management of bronchiectasis, including airway clearance techniques, pharmacological therapy, immunization, and smoking cessation, is essential to reduce symptoms, prevent exacerbations, and improve quality of life in affected individuals. By understanding the relationship between bronchiectasis and other respiratory conditions and addressing overlapping symptoms and comorbidities, healthcare providers can optimize outcomes and enhance the care of individuals living with bronchiectasis.

Recurrent Respiratory Infections: Understanding the Impact and Management

Recurrent respiratory infections (RRIs) represent a significant health concern characterized by multiple episodes of acute respiratory tract infections, including upper respiratory tract infections (URTIs) and lower respiratory tract infections (LRTIs). These infections pose a substantial burden on affected individuals, leading to morbidity, impaired quality of life, and potential complications. This section explores the epidemiology, risk factors, clinical presentation, diagnosis, management, and preventive strategies for recurrent respiratory infections.

Epidemiology and Burden of Recurrent Respiratory Infections:

Recurrent respiratory infections are common, particularly in children, older adults, and individuals with underlying comorbidities or immunocompromising conditions. The frequency and severity of RRIs may vary depending on factors such as age, immune status, environmental exposures, and healthcare utilization patterns. RRIs contribute significantly to healthcare utilization, including primary care visits, emergency department visits, and hospitalizations, placing a considerable economic burden on healthcare systems.

Risk Factors for Recurrent Respiratory Infections:

Several factors contribute to the development of recurrent respiratory infections, including:

- **Immunodeficiency:** Primary immunodeficiency disorders, secondary immunodeficiency states (e.g., HIV infection, immunosuppressive therapy), and functional immune defects predispose individuals to recurrent infections by impairing immune responses against respiratory pathogens.
- **Environmental Exposures:** Exposure to indoor and outdoor air pollutants, tobacco smoke, allergens, and occupational irritants can increase the risk of respiratory infections by compromising airway integrity and immune function.
- **Underlying Respiratory Conditions:** Individuals with chronic respiratory conditions such as asthma, COPD, bronchiectasis, or cystic fibrosis are at increased risk of recurrent respiratory infections due to impaired mucociliary clearance, airway inflammation, and structural lung damage.
- **Age:** Infants, young children, and older adults

are particularly vulnerable to recurrent respiratory infections due to age-related factors such as immature immune systems, waning immunity, and comorbidities.

Clinical Presentation of Recurrent Respiratory Infections:

The clinical presentation of recurrent respiratory infections varies depending on the underlying pathogens, affected anatomical sites, and immune status of the individual. Common symptoms of RRIs may include:

- **Upper Respiratory Tract Infections (URTIs):** Symptoms of URTIs include nasal congestion, rhinorrhea, sore throat, cough, sneezing, fever, and malaise. URTIs are typically caused by viruses such as rhinovirus, influenza virus, respiratory syncytial virus (RSV), adenovirus, or coronavirus.
- **Lower Respiratory Tract Infections (LRTIs):** LRTIs manifest as symptoms such as cough, sputum production, dyspnea, chest pain, fever, and systemic symptoms. LRTIs may be caused by viral pathogens (e.g., influenza, RSV) or bacterial pathogens (e.g., Streptococcus pneumoniae, Haemophilus influenzae, Mycoplasma pneumoniae).

Diagnosis of Recurrent Respiratory Infections:

The diagnosis of recurrent respiratory infections relies on clinical evaluation, including medical history, physical examination, and laboratory testing. Diagnostic tests may include:

- **Microbiological Testing:** Respiratory specimens (e.g., nasopharyngeal swabs, sputum samples) can be analyzed using molecular methods (e.g., polymerase chain reaction [PCR]) or culture-based techniques to identify viral or bacterial pathogens responsible for the infection.

- **Imaging Studies:** Chest X-rays or computed tomography (CT) scans may be performed to evaluate for signs of lower respiratory tract involvement, such as pneumonia or bronchiectasis, particularly in individuals with recurrent or severe respiratory infections.
- **Immunological Evaluation:** Immunological testing, including assessment of immunoglobulin levels, lymphocyte subsets, and specific antibody responses, may be indicated in individuals suspected of having underlying immunodeficiency disorders contributing to recurrent respiratory infections.

Management of Recurrent Respiratory Infections:

The management of recurrent respiratory infections focuses on symptom relief, prevention of complications, and reduction of recurrence rates. Key components of management include:

- **Pharmacological Therapy:** Antimicrobial agents may be prescribed for bacterial infections, while antiviral medications may be indicated for specific viral pathogens (e.g., influenza, herpes simplex virus). Symptomatic relief can be achieved with analgesics, antipyretics, cough suppressants, and expectorants.
- **Immunomodulatory Therapy:** Immunomodulatory agents, such as intravenous immunoglobulin (IVIG) or immunomodulators (e.g., interferon-gamma), may be considered in individuals with underlying immunodeficiency disorders or recurrent severe infections unresponsive to conventional therapies.
- **Airway Clearance Techniques:** Airway clearance techniques, including chest physiotherapy, postural drainage, percussion, and vibration, help mobilize and remove excess mucus from the airways, reducing the risk of infection and improving lung function in individuals with conditions such as bronchiectasis or cystic fibrosis.

- **Preventive Measures:** Vaccination against common respiratory pathogens, including influenza, pneumococcus, pertussis, and Haemophilus influenzae type b (Hib), is essential in reducing the risk of respiratory infections and preventing complications, particularly in high-risk populations such as young children, older adults, and individuals with chronic medical conditions.

Conclusion:

Recurrent respiratory infections pose a significant health burden, leading to morbidity, healthcare utilization, and impaired quality of life. Understanding the epidemiology, risk factors, clinical presentation, diagnosis, and management of recurrent respiratory infections is essential in optimizing outcomes and reducing recurrence rates in affected individuals. By implementing preventive measures, timely diagnosis, and evidence-based management strategies, healthcare providers can mitigate the impact of recurrent respiratory infections and improve the respiratory health and well-being of individuals at risk.

Pneumonia: Understanding a Common Respiratory Infection

Pneumonia is a prevalent respiratory infection characterized by inflammation of the lung parenchyma, typically caused by infectious agents such as bacteria, viruses, fungi, or parasites. This section explores the epidemiology, etiology, pathophysiology, clinical presentation, diagnosis, management, and prevention of pneumonia, highlighting its significant impact on public health and individual morbidity.

Epidemiology of Pneumonia:

Pneumonia is a leading cause of morbidity and mortality worldwide, affecting individuals of all ages, with particular vulnerability among young children, older adults, and individuals with underlying comorbidities or immunocompromised states. The incidence of pneumonia varies by geographic region, seasonality, and demographic factors, with higher rates observed in low-income countries and during winter months. Pneumonia accounts for a substantial burden of hospitalizations, healthcare costs, and premature deaths globally.

Etiology and Pathophysiology of Pneumonia:

Pneumonia can be caused by a wide range of infectious agents, including bacteria (e.g., Streptococcus pneumoniae, Haemophilus influenzae, Mycoplasma pneumoniae), viruses (e.g., influenza virus, respiratory syncytial virus [RSV], adenovirus), fungi (e.g., Pneumocystis jirovecii, Candida species), and less commonly, parasites (e.g., Pneumocystis carinii). The pathogenesis of pneumonia involves the inhalation or aspiration of infectious particles into the lower respiratory tract, leading to alveolar inflammation, consolidation, impaired gas exchange, and respiratory symptoms such as cough, fever, dyspnea, and chest pain.

Clinical Presentation and Diagnosis of Pneumonia:

The clinical presentation of pneumonia varies depending on the causative organism, underlying host factors, and disease severity. Common symptoms of pneumonia may include acute onset of fever, chills, productive cough, pleuritic chest pain, dyspnea, and systemic symptoms such as malaise, fatigue, and myalgias. Physical examination findings may reveal signs of respiratory distress, crackles, dullness to percussion, and bronchial breath sounds. Diagnostic evaluation of pneumonia typically involves:

- **Clinical Assessment:** Medical history, physical examination, and assessment of clinical symptoms and risk factors help guide the initial evaluation and management of suspected pneumonia.
- **Radiological Imaging:** Chest X-ray is the primary imaging modality for diagnosing pneumonia, demonstrating characteristic findings such as pulmonary infiltrates, lobar consolidation, and pleural effusions. Computed tomography (CT) scan may be performed in cases of suspected complicated or atypical pneumonia.
- **Microbiological Testing:** Respiratory specimens (e.g., sputum, nasopharyngeal swabs) can be analyzed using microbiological techniques such as culture, polymerase chain reaction (PCR), or antigen detection assays to identify the causative pathogen and guide targeted antimicrobial therapy.

Management of Pneumonia:

The management of pneumonia involves prompt initiation of antimicrobial therapy, supportive care, and targeted interventions to reduce complications and improve outcomes. Key components of pneumonia management include:

- **Antimicrobial Therapy:** Empirical antimicrobial therapy should be initiated promptly based on clinical suspicion and severity of illness, with selection guided by local antimicrobial resistance patterns and risk factors for specific pathogens. Antibiotic therapy may be adjusted based on microbiological results and clinical response.
- **Supportive Care:** Supportive measures such as supplemental oxygen therapy, hydration, analgesia, and antipyretics help alleviate symptoms, improve patient comfort, and facilitate recovery. Close monitoring of vital signs, oxygen saturation, and clinical status is essential

to assess treatment response and identify complications.
- **Respiratory Support:** In severe cases of pneumonia with respiratory failure or acute respiratory distress syndrome (ARDS), respiratory support may be necessary, including non-invasive ventilation or invasive mechanical ventilation in an intensive care setting.
- **Adjunctive Therapies:** Adjunctive therapies such as corticosteroids, bronchodilators, or antiviral agents may be considered in specific cases, particularly in individuals with severe or complicated pneumonia or underlying comorbidities.

Prevention of Pneumonia:

Preventive measures play a crucial role in reducing the burden of pneumonia and preventing transmission of infectious agents. Key preventive strategies include:

- **Vaccination:** Vaccination against common pathogens such as Streptococcus pneumoniae, influenza virus, and Haemophilus influenzae type b (Hib) is essential in preventing pneumonia, particularly in high-risk populations such as young children, older adults, and individuals with chronic medical conditions or immunocompromised states.
- **Hand Hygiene:** Practicing good hand hygiene, including regular handwashing with soap and water or alcohol-based hand sanitizers, helps reduce the spread of respiratory pathogens and prevent transmission of infections.
- **Smoking Cessation:** Smoking cessation is paramount in preventing pneumonia and reducing the risk of respiratory infections, as smoking impairs mucociliary clearance, weakens the immune response, and increases susceptibility to respiratory pathogens.
- **Environmental Hygiene:** Maintaining clean indoor air

quality, minimizing exposure to indoor and outdoor pollutants, and practicing respiratory hygiene measures (e.g., covering coughs and sneezes, disposing of tissues properly) help prevent the transmission of respiratory infections in community settings.

Conclusion:

Pneumonia is a common and potentially serious respiratory infection characterized by inflammation of the lung parenchyma, often caused by infectious agents such as bacteria, viruses, fungi, or parasites. Understanding the epidemiology, etiology, clinical presentation, diagnosis, management, and prevention of pneumonia is essential in reducing its impact on public health and individual morbidity. By implementing preventive measures, timely diagnosis, and evidence-based management strategies, healthcare providers can mitigate the burden of pneumonia and improve outcomes for affected individuals.

Pneumothorax: Understanding a Disruptive Pulmonary Condition

Pneumothorax is a potentially life-threatening condition characterized by the presence of air in the pleural space, leading to partial or complete collapse of the affected lung. This section provides an overview of pneumothorax, including its classification, etiology, clinical presentation, diagnosis, management, and potential complications.

Classification of Pneumothorax:

Pneumothorax can be classified into several categories based on its etiology, including:

1. **Primary Spontaneous Pneumothorax:** Occurs in the

absence of underlying lung disease, typically in young, otherwise healthy individuals, and is often associated with the rupture of small subpleural blebs or bullae.
2. **Secondary Spontaneous Pneumothorax:** Develops in individuals with underlying lung disease, such as chronic obstructive pulmonary disease (COPD), cystic fibrosis, interstitial lung disease, or malignancy, due to the rupture of pre-existing lung cysts, bullae, or lung parenchymal lesions.
3. **Traumatic Pneumothorax:** Results from chest trauma, such as blunt or penetrating injuries, rib fractures, or iatrogenic causes (e.g., central venous catheter insertion, thoracic surgery), leading to disruption of the pleural integrity and the entry of air into the pleural space.
4. **Tension Pneumothorax:** Represents a medical emergency characterized by progressive accumulation of air in the pleural space, leading to mediastinal shift, compression of the contralateral lung, and hemodynamic compromise. Tension pneumothorax can occur spontaneously or as a complication of trauma or mechanical ventilation.

Etiology and Pathophysiology:

The pathophysiology of pneumothorax involves the entry of air into the pleural space, disrupting the negative intrapleural pressure that maintains lung expansion and respiratory function. In primary spontaneous pneumothorax, the rupture of subpleural blebs or bullae, often located apically or along the lung periphery, allows air to escape from the alveoli into the pleural cavity. Secondary spontaneous pneumothorax occurs due to the rupture of pre-existing lung cysts or bullae associated with underlying lung disease. Traumatic pneumothorax results from chest trauma, leading to the disruption of pleural integrity and air entry into the pleural space.

Clinical Presentation:

The clinical presentation of pneumothorax varies depending on its severity, underlying etiology, and the presence of associated complications such as tension pneumothorax. Common symptoms of pneumothorax may include:

- **Sudden onset of pleuritic chest pain:** Sharp or stabbing chest pain, exacerbated by breathing or movement, is a hallmark symptom of pneumothorax and may radiate to the shoulder or back.
- **Dyspnea:** Shortness of breath or difficulty breathing may occur due to lung collapse and impaired gas exchange.
- **Tachypnea:** Rapid respiratory rate may be observed as a compensatory mechanism to maintain adequate ventilation.
- **Decreased breath sounds:** Auscultation of the chest may reveal diminished or absent breath sounds over the affected hemithorax.
- **Hypoxemia:** Decreased oxygen saturation may occur due to impaired gas exchange secondary to lung collapse.

Diagnosis of Pneumothorax:

The diagnosis of pneumothorax is based on a combination of clinical evaluation, radiological imaging, and diagnostic procedures. Key diagnostic modalities include:

- **Chest X-ray:** Chest X-ray is the initial imaging modality of choice for diagnosing pneumothorax, demonstrating characteristic findings such as visceral pleural line, absence of lung markings beyond the pleural line, and mediastinal shift in tension pneumothorax.
- **Computed Tomography (CT) Scan:** CT scan of the chest may be performed to evaluate the extent of lung collapse, identify underlying lung pathology, or

assess for complications such as pneumomediastinum or subcutaneous emphysema.
- **Ultrasound:** Point-of-care ultrasound is a valuable tool for diagnosing pneumothorax at the bedside, particularly in emergency settings, by visualizing the presence of pleural sliding or lung point.
- **Arterial Blood Gas (ABG) Analysis:** ABG analysis may reveal hypoxemia, respiratory alkalosis, or hypercapnia in individuals with pneumothorax, depending on the degree of lung collapse and gas exchange impairment.

Management of Pneumothorax:

The management of pneumothorax depends on its severity, underlying etiology, and associated complications. Treatment options may include:

- **Observation:** Small, asymptomatic pneumothoraces may be managed conservatively with observation and serial chest X-rays to monitor for resolution or progression.
- **Oxygen Therapy:** Supplemental oxygen therapy is indicated to improve oxygenation and reduce hypoxemia in individuals with pneumothorax, particularly those with significant lung collapse or respiratory distress.
- **Thoracostomy:** Thoracostomy, or chest tube placement, is the primary treatment for symptomatic or tension pneumothorax, allowing for the evacuation of air from the pleural space and re-expansion of the lung.
- **Needle Decompression:** Needle decompression may be performed as a temporizing measure in individuals with tension pneumothorax, using a large-bore needle or catheter inserted into the pleural space to relieve tension and restore hemodynamic stability.
- **Surgical Intervention:** Surgical intervention, such as video-assisted thoracoscopic surgery (VATS) or open

thoracotomy, may be indicated for recurrent or refractory pneumothorax, underlying lung pathology, or complications such as bronchopleural fistula.

Complications of Pneumothorax:

Complications of pneumothorax may include:

- **Tension Pneumothorax:** Tension pneumothorax represents a life-threatening complication characterized by progressive accumulation of air in the pleural space, leading to mediastinal shift, compression of the contralateral lung, and hemodynamic compromise.
- **Pneumomediastinum:** Pneumomediastinum occurs when air escapes from the pleural space into the mediastinum, leading to subcutaneous emphysema, chest pain, and dysphagia.
- **Bronchopleural Fistula:** Bronchopleural fistula is a communication between the bronchial tree and the pleural space, leading to persistent air leak, recurrent pneumothorax, and increased risk of infection.

Prevention of Pneumothorax:

Preventive measures to reduce the risk of pneumothorax include:

- **Smoking Cessation:** Smoking cessation is essential in preventing primary spontaneous pneumothorax and reducing the risk of lung disease associated with secondary spontaneous pneumothorax.
- **Occupational Safety:** Ensuring workplace safety measures, including proper use of protective equipment, minimizing exposure to occupational hazards, and adhering to safety protocols, helps prevent traumatic pneumothorax in high-risk occupations.
- **Education and Awareness:** Educating individuals about

the signs and symptoms of pneumothorax, risk factors, and preventive measures can help promote early recognition, prompt treatment, and improved outcomes.

Conclusion:

Pneumothorax is a potentially life-threatening condition characterized by the presence of air in the pleural space, leading to lung collapse and respiratory impairment. Understanding the classification, etiology, clinical presentation, diagnosis, management, and potential complications of pneumothorax is essential for healthcare providers to optimize patient care and outcomes. By implementing preventive measures, timely diagnosis, and evidence-based management strategies, healthcare providers can mitigate the impact of pneumothorax and improve the respiratory health and well-being of affected individuals.

Sleep Disordered Breathing: Understanding the Impact on Respiratory Health

Sleep-disordered breathing (SDB) encompasses a spectrum of respiratory disorders characterized by abnormal breathing patterns during sleep, ranging from snoring and upper airway resistance syndrome (UARS) to obstructive sleep apnea (OSA) and central sleep apnea (CSA). This section provides an overview of sleep-disordered breathing, including its classification, epidemiology, pathophysiology, clinical presentation, diagnosis, management, and potential complications.

Classification of Sleep Disordered Breathing:

Sleep-disordered breathing can be classified into several categories based on the underlying pathophysiology and predominant respiratory abnormalities:

1. **Obstructive Sleep Apnea (OSA):** OSA is characterized by recurrent episodes of complete or partial upper airway obstruction during sleep, leading to intermittent hypoxemia, hypercapnia, and sleep fragmentation.
2. **Central Sleep Apnea (CSA):** CSA involves periods of absent or decreased respiratory effort during sleep, resulting in pauses in breathing and impaired gas exchange, often associated with central nervous system dysfunction or underlying medical conditions.
3. **Mixed Sleep Apnea:** Mixed sleep apnea is characterized by a combination of obstructive and central respiratory events during sleep, presenting diagnostic and management challenges.
4. **Upper Airway Resistance Syndrome (UARS):** UARS is characterized by increased resistance to airflow during sleep, leading to recurrent arousals, fragmented sleep, and daytime symptoms such as excessive daytime sleepiness and fatigue.

Epidemiology of Sleep Disordered Breathing:

Sleep-disordered breathing is highly prevalent, particularly in middle-aged and older adults, with a higher prevalence observed in men compared to women. The prevalence of OSA varies by population and risk factors, with estimates ranging from 9% to 38% in adult populations. Risk factors for sleep-disordered breathing include obesity, male gender, advancing age, craniofacial abnormalities, alcohol consumption, smoking, and sedative medications.

Pathophysiology of Sleep Disordered Breathing:

The pathophysiology of sleep-disordered breathing involves complex interactions between anatomical, physiological, and neurological factors contributing to upper airway collapse, respiratory instability, and impaired ventilatory control during sleep. Key mechanisms implicated in sleep-disordered breathing include:

- **Upper Airway Anatomy:** Anatomical factors such as obesity, craniofacial abnormalities, enlarged tonsils, and retrognathia can predispose individuals to upper airway collapse and obstruction during sleep.
- **Pharyngeal Muscle Tone:** Decreased tone of the pharyngeal dilator muscles during sleep, particularly during rapid eye movement (REM) sleep, contributes to upper airway collapse and obstruction in individuals with sleep-disordered breathing.
- **Ventilatory Control:** Dysregulation of respiratory control mechanisms, including central and peripheral chemoreceptors, loop gain, and arousal threshold, can lead to abnormal breathing patterns and ventilatory instability during sleep.
- **Genetic Factors:** Genetic predisposition plays a role in the development of sleep-disordered breathing, with familial clustering observed in some cases, suggesting a genetic component to susceptibility.

Clinical Presentation of Sleep Disordered Breathing:

The clinical presentation of sleep-disordered breathing varies depending on the severity, type, and underlying comorbidities. Common symptoms of sleep-disordered breathing may include:

- **Snoring:** Loud, habitual snoring is a hallmark symptom of obstructive sleep apnea and may be accompanied by gasping or choking episodes during sleep.
- **Excessive Daytime Sleepiness:** Excessive daytime sleepiness, fatigue, and impaired concentration are common symptoms of sleep-disordered breathing, resulting from disrupted sleep architecture and recurrent arousals during the night.

- **Witnessed Apneas:** Witnessed apneas or choking episodes reported by bed partners or family members are indicative of significant respiratory disturbances during sleep.
- **Morning Headaches:** Morning headaches, dry mouth, and sore throat may occur due to nocturnal hypoxemia, hypercapnia, and upper airway irritation.
- **Nocturia:** Nocturnal polyuria and frequent awakenings to urinate may be present in individuals with sleep-disordered breathing due to increased sympathetic activity and altered fluid dynamics.

Diagnosis of Sleep Disordered Breathing:

The diagnosis of sleep-disordered breathing involves a combination of clinical evaluation, sleep history assessment, overnight polysomnography (PSG), and home sleep apnea testing (HSAT). Diagnostic criteria for sleep-disordered breathing include:

- **Polysomnography (PSG):** PSG is the gold standard diagnostic test for sleep-disordered breathing, providing comprehensive monitoring of physiological parameters such as airflow, respiratory effort, oxygen saturation, sleep stages, and arousals during overnight sleep.
- **Home Sleep Apnea Testing (HSAT):** HSAT may be used as an alternative to PSG for diagnosing uncomplicated obstructive sleep apnea in select individuals, offering convenience and cost-effectiveness for home-based testing.
- **Clinical Assessment:** Clinical evaluation by a sleep medicine specialist includes a comprehensive sleep history, physical examination, assessment of symptoms, and identification of risk factors for sleep-disordered breathing.

Management of Sleep Disordered Breathing:

The management of sleep-disordered breathing aims to improve symptoms, reduce cardiovascular risk, and enhance quality of life through a combination of behavioral interventions, positive airway pressure therapy, oral appliances, surgical procedures, and adjunctive therapies. Key components of management include:

- **Positive Airway Pressure (PAP) Therapy:** Continuous positive airway pressure (CPAP), bilevel positive airway pressure (BiPAP), or automatic positive airway pressure (APAP) therapy is the primary treatment for moderate to severe obstructive sleep apnea, providing pneumatic splinting of the upper airway and preventing collapse during sleep.
- **Oral Appliances:** Mandibular advancement devices (MADs) or tongue-retaining devices (TRDs) may be considered as alternative treatments for individuals with mild to moderate obstructive sleep apnea or those unable to tolerate PAP therapy.
- **Behavioral Interventions:** Behavioral interventions such as weight loss, dietary modifications, regular exercise, positional therapy, and avoidance of alcohol, sedatives, and tobacco can help reduce the severity of sleep-disordered breathing and improve treatment outcomes.
- **Surgical Procedures:** Surgical interventions, including uvulopalatopharyngoplasty (UPPP), tonsillectomy, adenoidectomy, septoplasty, and maxillomandibular advancement (MMA), may be considered in select cases of obstructive sleep apnea refractory to conservative measures or for correction of anatomical abnormalities contributing to upper airway obstruction.
- **Adjunctive Therapies:** Adjunctive therapies such as

positional therapy devices, nasal dilators, oropharyngeal exercises, and myofunctional therapy may be used in combination with PAP therapy or oral appliances to optimize treatment outcomes and adherence.

Complications of Sleep Disordered Breathing:

Untreated sleep-disordered breathing can lead to a wide range of complications, including:

- **Cardiovascular Disease:** Sleep-disordered breathing is associated with an increased risk of hypertension, coronary artery disease, stroke, arrhythmias, and heart failure, attributable to intermittent hypoxemia, sympathetic activation, and systemic inflammation.
- **Metabolic Dysfunction:** Sleep-disordered breathing is linked to metabolic disturbances such as insulin resistance, dyslipidemia, metabolic syndrome, and obesity, contributing to the development of type 2 diabetes and cardiovascular complications.
- **Neurocognitive Impairment:** Chronic sleep-disordered breathing is associated with neurocognitive deficits, including impaired attention, memory, executive function, and psychomotor performance, leading to decreased quality of life and functional impairment.
- **Daytime Functioning:** Excessive daytime sleepiness, fatigue, impaired concentration, and diminished psychosocial functioning are common consequences of untreated sleep-disordered breathing, affecting work productivity, driving safety, and interpersonal relationships.

Prevention of Sleep Disordered Breathing:

Preventive measures to reduce the risk of sleep-disordered breathing include:

- **Weight Management:** Weight loss and maintenance of a healthy body weight through diet and exercise play a crucial role in reducing the risk of sleep-disordered breathing, particularly in individuals with obesity or central adiposity.
- **Avoidance of Sedatives and Alcohol:** Limiting the use of sedative medications, hypnotics, and alcohol consumption, particularly before bedtime, helps minimize upper airway collapse and respiratory disturbances during sleep.
- **Sleep Hygiene:** Practicing good sleep hygiene habits, such as maintaining a regular sleep schedule, creating a comfortable sleep environment, and avoiding stimulating activities before bedtime, promotes restorative sleep and reduces the risk of sleep-disordered breathing.
- **Screening and Early Intervention:** Screening individuals at risk for sleep-disordered breathing, such as those with obesity, snoring, witnessed apneas, or daytime sleepiness, allows for early detection and intervention, improving treatment outcomes and reducing complications.

Conclusion:

Sleep-disordered breathing encompasses a spectrum of respiratory disorders characterized by abnormal breathing patterns during sleep, ranging from snoring and upper airway resistance syndrome to obstructive and central sleep apnea. Understanding the classification, epidemiology, pathophysiology, clinical presentation, diagnosis, management, and potential complications of sleep-disordered breathing is essential for healthcare providers to optimize patient care and outcomes. By implementing preventive measures, timely diagnosis, and evidence-based management strategies, healthcare providers can mitigate the impact of sleep-disordered breathing and improve the respiratory health and quality of life of affected individuals.

Psychological Impacts of Respiratory Disorders: Understanding the Interplay

Respiratory disorders, ranging from asthma to chronic obstructive pulmonary disease (COPD) and sleep-disordered breathing, can exert profound psychological effects on individuals, influencing their emotional well-being, quality of life, and mental health. This section delves into the psychological impacts of respiratory disorders, exploring their prevalence, etiology, clinical manifestations, assessment, management, and implications for holistic patient care.

Prevalence and Burden:

The prevalence of psychological comorbidities in individuals with respiratory disorders is significant, with studies reporting high rates of anxiety, depression, stress, and impaired quality of life among affected individuals. The burden of psychological symptoms is particularly pronounced in chronic and severe respiratory conditions, such as severe asthma, COPD exacerbations, and advanced stages of respiratory failure.

Etiology and Mechanisms:

The etiology of psychological comorbidities in respiratory disorders is multifactorial, involving complex interactions between biological, psychological, and social determinants. Key contributing factors include:

- **Disease Severity:** The severity of respiratory symptoms, functional impairment, and disease progression can exacerbate psychological distress and negatively impact

mental health outcomes.
- **Chronicity and Uncertainty:** Living with a chronic respiratory condition characterized by unpredictable symptoms, exacerbations, and treatment challenges can lead to feelings of helplessness, frustration, and anxiety about the future.
- **Social Isolation:** Social isolation, stigma, and impaired social functioning due to respiratory symptoms or mobility limitations can contribute to loneliness, depression, and reduced quality of life.
- **Biological Pathways:** Biological mechanisms underlying respiratory disorders, such as chronic inflammation, oxidative stress, hypoxemia, and altered neurotransmitter signaling, may also influence mood regulation, cognitive function, and emotional well-being.

Clinical Manifestations:

The clinical manifestations of psychological comorbidities in respiratory disorders encompass a broad spectrum of symptoms, including:

- **Anxiety:** Anxiety symptoms, such as excessive worry, restlessness, palpitations, and hyperventilation, are common in individuals with respiratory disorders, particularly during acute exacerbations or episodes of breathlessness.
- **Depression:** Depressive symptoms, such as sadness, loss of interest or pleasure, fatigue, sleep disturbances, and changes in appetite or weight, are prevalent among individuals with chronic respiratory conditions, contributing to impaired quality of life and functional impairment.
- **Stress and Coping:** Chronic stress, maladaptive coping strategies, and emotional dysregulation are common responses to the challenges of living with a respiratory

disorder, leading to heightened physiological arousal, cognitive distortions, and interpersonal difficulties.
- **Psychosocial Impact:** Respiratory disorders can exert a significant psychosocial impact on individuals and their families, affecting relationships, work performance, financial stability, and social participation, thereby exacerbating feelings of isolation, burden, and distress.

Assessment and Screening:

The assessment and screening of psychological comorbidities in individuals with respiratory disorders are essential for comprehensive patient care and treatment planning. Key considerations include:

- **Comprehensive Evaluation:** A comprehensive evaluation of psychological symptoms, functional impairment, and quality of life is integral to identifying individuals at risk for psychological comorbidities and tailoring interventions to their specific needs.
- **Screening Tools:** Validated screening tools, such as the Hospital Anxiety and Depression Scale (HADS), Beck Depression Inventory (BDI), Generalized Anxiety Disorder 7-item scale (GAD-7), and Patient Health Questionnaire-9 (PHQ-9), can be used to assess the severity of anxiety, depression, and related symptoms in individuals with respiratory disorders.
- **Multidisciplinary Collaboration:** Multidisciplinary collaboration between respiratory specialists, primary care providers, mental health professionals, and social support services facilitates comprehensive assessment, integrated care planning, and coordinated management of psychological comorbidities in individuals with respiratory disorders.

Management Strategies:

The management of psychological comorbidities in individuals with respiratory disorders involves a multimodal approach targeting symptom relief, functional improvement, and holistic well-being. Key strategies include:

- **Psychoeducation:** Providing individuals with information about their respiratory condition, treatment options, self-management strategies, and coping skills empowers them to actively participate in their care and improve treatment adherence.
- **Cognitive-Behavioral Therapy (CBT):** CBT is a evidence-based psychotherapy approach that targets maladaptive thought patterns, behavioral responses, and coping strategies associated with anxiety, depression, and stress in individuals with respiratory disorders, promoting adaptive coping and symptom management.
- **Mindfulness and Relaxation Techniques:** Mindfulness-based interventions, relaxation techniques, and stress management strategies, such as deep breathing exercises, progressive muscle relaxation, and guided imagery, can help individuals reduce physiological arousal, enhance emotional regulation, and improve sleep quality.
- **Social Support:** Social support networks, peer support groups, and community resources play a crucial role in providing emotional support, practical assistance, and social engagement for individuals with respiratory disorders, reducing feelings of isolation and enhancing coping resilience.
- **Medication Management:** Pharmacological interventions, such as antidepressants, anxiolytics, and psychotropic medications, may be indicated for individuals with moderate to severe psychological symptoms or comorbid psychiatric disorders, under the guidance of a mental health professional.

Implications for Holistic Patient Care:

Recognizing and addressing the psychological impact of respiratory disorders is essential for providing holistic patient-centered care and optimizing health outcomes. Integrating psychological assessment, supportive interventions, and collaborative care into respiratory management plans can improve treatment adherence, symptom control, and quality of life for individuals with respiratory disorders.

Conclusion:

The psychological impact of respiratory disorders extends beyond the physical manifestations of disease, encompassing a wide range of emotional, cognitive, and psychosocial factors that influence individual well-being, quality of life, and treatment outcomes. Understanding the prevalence, etiology, clinical manifestations, assessment, management, and implications of psychological comorbidities in respiratory disorders is essential for healthcare providers to deliver comprehensive, patient-centered care and support individuals in managing their respiratory health and overall well-being. By addressing the psychological needs of individuals with respiratory disorders, healthcare providers can enhance treatment adherence, promote adaptive coping, and improve overall health outcomes for affected individuals.

CHAPTER 7: ADVANCES IN RESEARCH AND FUTURE DIRECTIONS

Exploring Emerging Therapeutic Targets for Respiratory Disorders

As our understanding of respiratory disorders evolves, so does the quest for novel therapeutic targets to address unmet needs, improve treatment outcomes, and enhance patient care. This section delves into the realm of emerging therapeutic targets for respiratory disorders, including asthma, chronic obstructive pulmonary disease (COPD), and other respiratory conditions, exploring promising avenues of research, innovative treatment modalities, and potential implications for future clinical practice.

1. Targeting Inflammatory Pathways:

Inflammatory processes play a central role in the pathogenesis of respiratory disorders, driving airway inflammation, bronchospasm, mucus hypersecretion, and tissue remodeling. Emerging therapeutic targets aim to modulate inflammatory pathways through various mechanisms, including:

- **Biologics:** Monoclonal antibodies targeting specific inflammatory mediators, such as interleukins (ILs), tumor necrosis factor-alpha (TNF-α), and eosinophils, offer targeted therapy for severe asthma and eosinophilic COPD, reducing exacerbations and improving lung function.
- **Small Molecule Inhibitors:** Small molecule inhibitors targeting intracellular signaling pathways, such as Janus kinase (JAK) inhibitors, phosphodiesterase (PDE) inhibitors, and tyrosine kinase inhibitors, show promise in modulating inflammatory responses and bronchodilator effects in asthma and COPD.
- **Anti-inflammatory Agents:** Novel anti-inflammatory agents, including cytokine inhibitors, Toll-like receptor (TLR) agonists, and nuclear factor-kappa B (NF-κB) inhibitors, hold potential for reducing airway inflammation, oxidative stress, and remodeling in respiratory disorders.

2. Enhancing Airway Smooth Muscle Function:

Abnormalities in airway smooth muscle function contribute to bronchospasm, airway hyperresponsiveness, and airflow limitation in respiratory disorders. Emerging therapeutic targets aim to modulate airway smooth muscle tone and contractility through various approaches, including:

- **Bronchodilators:** Next-generation bronchodilators targeting novel receptors, ion channels, or signaling pathways offer improved efficacy, duration of action, and selectivity for smooth muscle relaxation in asthma and COPD.
- **Antifibrotic Agents:** Antifibrotic agents targeting fibroblast activation, extracellular matrix deposition,

and myofibroblast differentiation hold promise for preventing airway remodeling, fibrosis, and smooth muscle hypertrophy in severe asthma and COPD.
- **Neurotransmitter Modulators:** Neurotransmitter modulators targeting neural pathways involved in airway smooth muscle contraction, such as acetylcholine, substance P, and neurokinins, offer potential for bronchodilation and symptom relief in respiratory disorders.

3. Restoring Epithelial Barrier Function:

Disruption of the airway epithelial barrier contributes to increased permeability, mucus production, and susceptibility to respiratory infections in respiratory disorders. Emerging therapeutic targets aim to restore epithelial barrier function and enhance mucociliary clearance through various strategies, including:

- **Mucolytic Agents:** Novel mucolytic agents targeting mucus viscosity, composition, and clearance mechanisms offer potential for reducing mucus plugging, airway obstruction, and exacerbations in asthma, COPD, and cystic fibrosis.
- **Epithelial Repair Stimulators:** Epithelial repair stimulators targeting growth factors, cell signaling pathways, and stem cell populations hold promise for promoting epithelial regeneration, wound healing, and barrier integrity in respiratory disorders.
- **Mucus Modulators:** Mucus modulators targeting mucin production, secretion, and rheological properties offer potential for optimizing airway hydration, clearance, and defense mechanisms against pathogens in respiratory disorders.

4. Personalized Medicine Approaches:

Advances in omics technologies, biomarker discovery, and precision medicine offer opportunities for personalized therapeutic interventions tailored to individual patient characteristics, disease phenotypes, and treatment responses. Emerging strategies include:

- **Biomarker-Guided Therapy:** Biomarker-guided approaches utilizing biomarkers of inflammation, oxidative stress, airway remodeling, and treatment response enable targeted therapy selection, dose optimization, and monitoring in asthma and COPD.
- **Genomic Medicine:** Genomic medicine approaches, including pharmacogenomics, gene editing, and gene therapy, hold promise for identifying genetic determinants of treatment response, developing gene-based therapies, and predicting disease progression in respiratory disorders.
- **Biomechanical Modeling:** Computational modeling techniques, such as finite element analysis, fluid dynamics simulation, and virtual airway reconstruction, enable personalized assessment of airway mechanics, airflow distribution, and treatment efficacy in respiratory disorders.

5. Novel Drug Delivery Systems:

Innovative drug delivery systems offer opportunities for targeted drug delivery, enhanced drug stability, and improved patient adherence in respiratory disorders. Emerging technologies include:

- **Nanomedicine:** Nanoparticle-based drug delivery systems, liposomal formulations, and nanoencapsulation strategies enable targeted delivery of therapeutic agents to the airways, reducing systemic side effects and improving treatment efficacy in respiratory

disorders.
- **Inhaler Devices:** Next-generation inhaler devices incorporating smart technology, electronic monitoring, and feedback mechanisms optimize inhalation technique, medication adherence, and disease management in asthma and COPD.
- **Implantable Devices:** Implantable drug delivery devices, such as bronchial stents, drug-eluting implants, and sustained-release platforms, offer localized delivery of therapeutic agents to the airways, facilitating long-term treatment adherence and symptom control in severe respiratory disorders.

Conclusion:

Emerging therapeutic targets for respiratory disorders offer promising avenues for advancing disease management, improving treatment outcomes, and enhancing patient care in asthma, COPD, and other respiratory conditions. By harnessing the potential of novel pharmacological agents, biotechnological innovations, personalized medicine approaches, and drug delivery systems, healthcare providers can optimize therapeutic interventions, address unmet clinical needs, and improve the respiratory health and quality of life of affected individuals. Collaborative research efforts, interdisciplinary collaboration, and translational approaches are essential for translating emerging therapeutic targets into clinical practice and realizing the full potential of precision medicine in respiratory care.

Precision Medicine Approaches in Respiratory Disorders: Optimizing Patient Care

Precision medicine, also known as personalized medicine, is revolutionizing the field of respiratory medicine by tailoring treatment strategies to individual patient characteristics, genetic makeup, disease phenotypes, and treatment responses. This section explores the principles, applications, challenges, and future directions of precision medicine approaches in respiratory disorders, including asthma, chronic obstructive pulmonary disease (COPD), cystic fibrosis, and pulmonary fibrosis.

1. Principles of Precision Medicine:

Precision medicine approaches in respiratory disorders are grounded in several key principles:

- **Individualized Treatment:** Precision medicine aims to tailor treatment strategies to the unique characteristics and needs of each patient, optimizing therapeutic efficacy, minimizing adverse effects, and improving treatment adherence.
- **Genomic Profiling:** Genomic profiling involves the analysis of genetic variants, gene expression patterns, and epigenetic modifications to identify genetic determinants of disease susceptibility, treatment response, and prognosis in respiratory disorders.
- **Biomarker Discovery:** Biomarker discovery encompasses the identification and validation of biomarkers, including blood markers, imaging biomarkers, and molecular signatures, to stratify patients based on disease severity, phenotypic characteristics, and treatment response.
- **Predictive Modeling:** Predictive modeling techniques, such as machine learning, artificial intelligence, and mathematical modeling, enable the development of predictive algorithms for forecasting disease progression, treatment outcomes, and personalized treatment recommendations.

2. Applications of Precision Medicine:

Precision medicine approaches have diverse applications in respiratory disorders, including:

- **Phenotypic Characterization:** Precision medicine enables the precise phenotypic characterization of respiratory disorders based on clinical, physiological, and molecular parameters, facilitating targeted therapy selection and individualized treatment planning.
- **Biomarker-Guided Therapy:** Biomarker-guided approaches utilize biomarkers of inflammation, oxidative stress, airway remodeling, and treatment response to guide therapeutic decision-making, optimize treatment efficacy, and monitor disease progression in respiratory disorders.
- **Genomic Medicine:** Genomic medicine approaches, including pharmacogenomics, gene editing, and gene therapy, leverage genetic information to identify genetic determinants of treatment response, develop gene-based therapies, and predict disease trajectories in respiratory disorders.
- **Personalized Drug Therapy:** Personalized drug therapy involves tailoring pharmacological interventions to individual patient characteristics, including genetic polymorphisms, biomarker profiles, and comorbidities, to optimize treatment outcomes and minimize adverse effects in respiratory disorders.

3. Challenges and Considerations:

Despite the promise of precision medicine in respiratory disorders, several challenges and considerations must be addressed:

- **Data Integration:** Integrating diverse sources of data,

including clinical data, genetic data, imaging data, and environmental factors, poses challenges for data standardization, interoperability, and integration into clinical workflows.
- **Ethical and Legal Issues:** Ethical considerations surrounding patient privacy, data security, informed consent, and data sharing require careful attention to ensure patient confidentiality, transparency, and compliance with regulatory guidelines.
- **Cost and Accessibility:** The cost of genomic sequencing, biomarker testing, and advanced imaging modalities may limit the accessibility of precision medicine approaches, particularly in resource-limited settings and underserved populations.
- **Clinical Implementation:** Translating precision medicine approaches from research laboratories to clinical practice requires interdisciplinary collaboration, clinician education, and infrastructure support to ensure successful implementation and integration into routine patient care.

4. Future Directions:

The future of precision medicine in respiratory disorders holds exciting opportunities for innovation and advancement, including:

- **Multiomics Integration:** Integrating multiomics data, including genomics, transcriptomics, proteomics, metabolomics, and microbiomics, enables comprehensive molecular profiling of respiratory disorders, facilitating precision diagnosis, treatment selection, and disease monitoring.
- **Digital Health Technologies:** Digital health technologies, such as wearable sensors, mobile health apps, and telemedicine platforms, offer opportunities

for remote monitoring, real-time data collection, and personalized interventions in respiratory disorders.
- **Patient Engagement:** Empowering patients as active participants in their care through patient education, shared decision-making, and personalized treatment plans fosters patient engagement, adherence, and satisfaction with precision medicine approaches in respiratory disorders.
- **Collaborative Research:** Collaborative research initiatives, consortia, and clinical trials facilitate large-scale data sharing, collaborative analysis, and validation of precision medicine approaches across diverse patient populations and healthcare settings.

Conclusion:

Precision medicine approaches hold transformative potential for revolutionizing the diagnosis, treatment, and management of respiratory disorders, ushering in an era of personalized, patient-centered care. By leveraging genomic profiling, biomarker discovery, predictive modeling, and personalized drug therapy, precision medicine enables healthcare providers to tailor treatment strategies to individual patient characteristics, optimize therapeutic efficacy, and improve patient outcomes in respiratory disorders. Despite challenges and considerations, the future of precision medicine in respiratory disorders is bright, with opportunities for innovation, collaboration, and advancements in clinical practice. By embracing precision medicine approaches, healthcare providers can enhance the respiratory health and quality of life of individuals affected by respiratory disorders, realizing the vision of personalized medicine in respiratory care.

Exploring Novel Diagnostic Techniques for Respiratory

Disorders

In the realm of respiratory medicine, diagnostic accuracy is paramount for guiding treatment decisions, monitoring disease progression, and optimizing patient outcomes. This section explores cutting-edge diagnostic techniques revolutionizing the field of respiratory medicine, including advancements in imaging modalities, biomarker analysis, physiological assessments, and digital health technologies.

1. Advanced Imaging Modalities:

Advancements in imaging modalities offer unprecedented insights into the structure, function, and pathology of the respiratory system, enabling early detection, accurate diagnosis, and personalized treatment planning. Key advancements include:

- **High-Resolution Computed Tomography (HRCT):** HRCT provides detailed imaging of the lung parenchyma, airways, and pulmonary vasculature, facilitating the diagnosis and characterization of interstitial lung diseases, pulmonary nodules, and bronchiectasis with high spatial resolution and minimal radiation exposure.
- **Magnetic Resonance Imaging (MRI):** MRI offers non-invasive imaging of the respiratory system, including assessment of lung perfusion, ventilation, and tissue composition, without the need for ionizing radiation, making it particularly valuable for evaluating lung cancer, pulmonary embolism, and congenital lung anomalies.
- **Positron Emission Tomography (PET):** PET imaging with radiopharmaceutical tracers, such as fluorodeoxyglucose (FDG), allows for metabolic imaging of lung tumors, mediastinal lymph nodes, and distant metastases, facilitating staging, treatment response assessment, and prognostic evaluation in lung cancer.

2. Biomarker Analysis:

Biomarker analysis offers a non-invasive approach for diagnosing, monitoring, and prognosticating respiratory disorders, providing valuable insights into disease pathogenesis, treatment response, and personalized medicine. Key advancements include:

- **Liquid Biopsies:** Liquid biopsy techniques, such as circulating tumor DNA (ctDNA), circulating tumor cells (CTCs), and exosomal RNA, enable minimally invasive detection of genetic mutations, epigenetic alterations, and biomarker profiles in respiratory malignancies, guiding treatment selection and monitoring for disease recurrence.
- **Exhaled Breath Analysis:** Exhaled breath analysis, utilizing volatile organic compounds (VOCs), exhaled nitric oxide (FeNO), and breath condensate biomarkers, offers a non-invasive approach for diagnosing asthma, chronic obstructive pulmonary disease (COPD), and other respiratory disorders, providing insights into airway inflammation, oxidative stress, and disease activity.
- **Biomarker Panels:** Multiplex biomarker panels, combining multiple analytes, such as cytokines, chemokines, and growth factors, enable comprehensive profiling of inflammatory, fibrotic, and immunomodulatory pathways in respiratory disorders, facilitating disease stratification, treatment response prediction, and personalized medicine approaches.

3. Physiological Assessments:

Physiological assessments provide valuable information about respiratory function, mechanics, and gas exchange, aiding in the diagnosis, monitoring, and management of respiratory disorders. Key advancements include:

- **Lung Function Testing:** Advanced lung function testing, including spirometry, plethysmography, diffusing capacity (DLCO), and impulse oscillometry (IOS), enables comprehensive evaluation of airflow limitation, lung volumes, gas exchange, and airway resistance in respiratory disorders, guiding treatment decisions and assessing disease severity.
- **Cardiopulmonary Exercise Testing (CPET):** CPET combines exercise testing with simultaneous measurement of cardiopulmonary parameters, including oxygen consumption (VO2), carbon dioxide production (VCO2), and ventilatory efficiency, providing insights into exercise capacity, functional impairment, and cardiovascular-pulmonary interactions in respiratory disorders, such as pulmonary hypertension and exercise-induced dyspnea.
- **Sleep Studies:** Polysomnography (PSG) and home sleep apnea testing (HSAT) enable comprehensive evaluation of sleep architecture, respiratory events, and nocturnal oxygenation, aiding in the diagnosis and management of sleep-disordered breathing, including obstructive sleep apnea (OSA), central sleep apnea (CSA), and sleep-related hypoventilation disorders.

4. Digital Health Technologies:

Digital health technologies offer innovative solutions for remote monitoring, real-time data collection, and personalized interventions in respiratory disorders, enhancing patient engagement, adherence, and self-management. Key advancements include:

- **Telemedicine and Remote Monitoring:** Telemedicine platforms, virtual visits, and remote monitoring devices enable remote consultation, symptom tracking, and treatment optimization for patients with respiratory

disorders, particularly in underserved areas or during public health crises, such as the COVID-19 pandemic.
- **Mobile Health Apps:** Mobile health apps, wearable sensors, and smart devices empower patients to monitor symptoms, track medication adherence, and participate in self-management strategies for respiratory disorders, fostering patient engagement, empowerment, and shared decision-making.
- **Artificial Intelligence (AI) and Machine Learning:** AI-driven algorithms, machine learning models, and predictive analytics enable data-driven decision-making, risk stratification, and personalized treatment recommendations for patients with respiratory disorders, leveraging large-scale datasets, electronic health records (EHRs), and clinical imaging data for precision medicine approaches.

Conclusion:

Novel diagnostic techniques in respiratory medicine, including advanced imaging modalities, biomarker analysis, physiological assessments, and digital health technologies, are revolutionizing the landscape of respiratory care, enabling early detection, accurate diagnosis, and personalized treatment planning for patients with respiratory disorders. By embracing these advancements, healthcare providers can improve diagnostic accuracy, enhance patient outcomes, and transform the delivery of respiratory care in the era of precision medicine. Collaborative research efforts, interdisciplinary collaboration, and technology integration are essential for realizing the full potential of these novel diagnostic techniques and optimizing respiratory health for individuals worldwide.

Immunotherapy Developments in Respiratory Disorders: A

Paradigm Shift in Treatment

Immunotherapy has emerged as a groundbreaking treatment modality in respiratory disorders, offering targeted interventions to modulate immune responses, reduce airway inflammation, and improve disease control. This section explores recent advancements in immunotherapy developments across various respiratory conditions, including asthma, allergic rhinitis, chronic obstructive pulmonary disease (COPD), and autoimmune lung diseases.

1. Allergen-Specific Immunotherapy (AIT) for Allergic Respiratory Disorders:

Allergen-specific immunotherapy (AIT), also known as allergy shots or desensitization therapy, is a cornerstone treatment for allergic respiratory disorders, including allergic asthma and allergic rhinitis. Recent developments in AIT include:

- **Subcutaneous Immunotherapy (SCIT):** Traditional SCIT involves the subcutaneous administration of allergen extracts, gradually increasing doses over time to induce tolerance and reduce allergic symptoms. Recent advances in SCIT formulations, including modified allergen extracts, adjuvants, and depot formulations, aim to enhance efficacy, safety, and convenience for patients.
- **Sublingual Immunotherapy (SLIT):** SLIT involves the sublingual administration of allergen extracts in liquid or tablet formulations, providing a convenient and well-tolerated alternative to SCIT. Recent developments in SLIT formulations, including standardized extracts, fast-dissolving tablets, and novel adjuvants, aim to optimize treatment outcomes and adherence in allergic respiratory disorders.
- **Component-Resolved Diagnosis (CRD):** CRD involves the identification and characterization of specific allergenic

components, such as proteins or peptides, responsible for allergic sensitization in individual patients. Recent developments in CRD technologies, including microarray assays, multiplex immunoassays, and recombinant allergen components, enable personalized AIT based on precise allergen recognition and targeted immune modulation.

2. Biologic Therapies for Severe Asthma:

Biologic therapies targeting specific inflammatory pathways have revolutionized the management of severe asthma, offering personalized treatment options for patients with uncontrolled symptoms despite standard therapy. Recent developments in biologic therapies for severe asthma include:

- **Anti-Interleukin-5 (IL-5) Agents:** Monoclonal antibodies targeting IL-5, such as mepolizumab, reslizumab, and benralizumab, selectively deplete eosinophils and suppress eosinophilic inflammation in severe asthma, reducing exacerbations, improving lung function, and enhancing quality of life.
- **Anti-Interleukin-4/13 (IL-4/13) Agents:** Monoclonal antibodies targeting IL-4 and IL-13, such as dupilumab, inhibit type 2 inflammatory responses, including eosinophilic inflammation, airway hyperresponsiveness, and IgE production, offering therapeutic benefits in severe asthma phenotypes characterized by type 2 inflammation.
- **Other Biologic Targets:** Emerging biologic targets in severe asthma include thymic stromal lymphopoietin (TSLP), interleukin-33 (IL-33), and prostaglandin D2 (PGD2), which play key roles in orchestrating type 2 immune responses, airway remodeling, and bronchial smooth muscle contraction, offering potential targets for future biologic therapies.

3. Immunomodulatory Therapies for COPD and Autoimmune Lung Diseases:

Immunomodulatory therapies targeting inflammatory pathways have shown promise in the treatment of chronic obstructive pulmonary disease (COPD) and autoimmune lung diseases, such as idiopathic pulmonary fibrosis (IPF) and connective tissue disease-associated interstitial lung disease (CTD-ILD). Recent developments in immunomodulatory therapies include:

- **Phosphodiesterase-4 (PDE4) Inhibitors:** PDE4 inhibitors, such as roflumilast, inhibit the breakdown of cyclic adenosine monophosphate (cAMP), reducing inflammation and exacerbations in COPD by inhibiting pro-inflammatory cytokine production and neutrophilic inflammation.
- **Tyrosine Kinase Inhibitors (TKIs):** TKIs, such as nintedanib and pirfenidone, target fibroblast activation, extracellular matrix deposition, and myofibroblast differentiation in IPF and CTD-ILD, slowing disease progression and improving survival in patients with progressive fibrotic lung diseases.
- **Anti-Inflammatory Agents:** Novel anti-inflammatory agents, including cytokine inhibitors, chemokine receptor antagonists, and JAK inhibitors, are under investigation for their potential role in modulating immune responses, reducing inflammation, and improving outcomes in COPD, IPF, and autoimmune lung diseases.

4. Vaccine Therapies for Respiratory Infections:

Vaccine therapies play a critical role in preventing respiratory infections, including influenza, pneumococcal pneumonia, and respiratory syncytial virus (RSV) infections, particularly in high-risk populations, such as children, older adults, and individuals with chronic respiratory diseases. Recent developments in vaccine therapies include:

- **Influenza Vaccines:** Seasonal influenza vaccines are routinely recommended for individuals with chronic respiratory diseases, such as asthma and COPD, to reduce the risk of influenza-related complications, hospitalizations, and exacerbations. Recent advancements in influenza vaccine technology, including adjuvanted, high-dose, and recombinant vaccines, aim to enhance vaccine efficacy and immunogenicity in high-risk populations.
- **Pneumococcal Vaccines:** Pneumococcal vaccines, including pneumococcal conjugate vaccines (PCV) and pneumococcal polysaccharide vaccines (PPSV), are recommended for individuals with chronic respiratory diseases, such as COPD and bronchiectasis, to prevent pneumococcal pneumonia, bacteremia, and invasive pneumococcal disease. Recent developments in pneumococcal vaccine formulations, including expanded serotype coverage and novel adjuvants, aim to improve vaccine effectiveness and durability in high-risk populations.
- **RSV Vaccines:** RSV vaccines are under development for the prevention of respiratory syncytial virus (RSV) infections in infants, young children, and older adults, particularly those with chronic respiratory diseases, such as bronchopulmonary dysplasia (BPD), cystic fibrosis (CF), and immunocompromised conditions. Recent advancements in RSV vaccine candidates, including live attenuated, subunit, and nanoparticle vaccines, aim to induce robust immune responses and provide durable protection against RSV infection and disease.

Conclusion:

Immunotherapy developments in respiratory disorders represent a paradigm shift in treatment paradigms, offering targeted interventions to modulate immune responses, reduce airway inflammation, and improve disease control. By leveraging advancements in allergen-specific immunotherapy, biologic therapies, immunomodulatory agents, and vaccine technologies, healthcare providers can optimize treatment outcomes, enhance patient quality of life, and transform the management of respiratory disorders in the era of precision medicine. Collaborative research efforts, interdisciplinary collaboration, and patient-centered care are essential for realizing the full potential of immunotherapy developments and improving respiratory health outcomes for individuals worldwide.

Advancements in Biomarker Identification for Respiratory Disorders

Biomarkers play a pivotal role in the diagnosis, prognosis, treatment selection, and monitoring of respiratory disorders, providing valuable insights into disease pathogenesis, severity, and treatment response. This section explores recent advancements in biomarker identification for various respiratory conditions, including asthma, chronic obstructive pulmonary disease (COPD), interstitial lung diseases (ILDs), and lung cancer, highlighting novel biomarkers, emerging technologies, and their potential clinical applications.

1. Asthma Biomarkers:

Asthma is a heterogeneous respiratory condition characterized by airway inflammation, bronchial hyperresponsiveness, and variable airflow obstruction. Biomarkers play a crucial role in phenotyping asthma, guiding treatment decisions, and monitoring disease activity. Recent advancements in asthma biomarker identification include:

- **Inflammatory Biomarkers:** Inflammatory biomarkers, such as fractional exhaled nitric oxide (FeNO), eosinophil counts, and cytokines (e.g., interleukins), reflect airway inflammation and guide the selection of anti-inflammatory therapies, such as inhaled corticosteroids (ICS) and biologic agents targeting specific inflammatory pathways (e.g., anti-IL-5 therapies).
- **Type 2 Biomarkers:** Biomarkers associated with type 2 inflammation, including periostin, serum IgE levels, and blood eosinophil counts, help identify patients with eosinophilic asthma and predict response to biologic therapies targeting type 2 immune pathways (e.g., anti-IL-4/13 and anti-IL-5 therapies).
- **Exhaled Breath Biomarkers:** Exhaled breath biomarkers, such as volatile organic compounds (VOCs), exhaled breath condensate (EBC) biomarkers, and breath metabolites, offer non-invasive insights into airway inflammation, oxidative stress, and lipid peroxidation in asthma, enabling personalized treatment approaches and disease monitoring.

2. COPD Biomarkers:

COPD is a progressive respiratory condition characterized by airflow limitation, chronic bronchitis, and emphysema, often associated with systemic inflammation and comorbidities. Biomarkers play a crucial role in diagnosing COPD, assessing disease severity, and predicting exacerbations. Recent advancements in COPD biomarker identification include:

- **Inflammatory Biomarkers:** Inflammatory biomarkers, such as C-reactive protein (CRP), fibrinogen, and interleukins (e.g., IL-6, IL-8), reflect systemic inflammation and predict COPD exacerbations,

hospitalizations, and disease progression, guiding treatment strategies and risk stratification in COPD patients.
- **Lung Function Biomarkers:** Biomarkers associated with lung function decline, such as lung function tests (e.g., spirometry, diffusing capacity), lung imaging (e.g., CT scans, MRI), and airflow limitation indices (e.g., FEV1/FVC ratio), help assess disease severity, monitor disease progression, and guide therapeutic interventions in COPD.
- **Biomarkers of Comorbidities:** Biomarkers associated with COPD-related comorbidities, such as cardiovascular disease (e.g., troponin, brain natriuretic peptide), osteoporosis (e.g., vitamin D levels, bone turnover markers), and depression/anxiety (e.g., serotonin, cortisol), aid in identifying and managing comorbid conditions, improving overall patient outcomes in COPD.

3. Interstitial Lung Disease (ILD) Biomarkers:

ILD encompasses a diverse group of diffuse parenchymal lung diseases characterized by inflammation, fibrosis, and impaired gas exchange. Biomarkers play a critical role in diagnosing ILD, assessing disease activity, and predicting prognosis. Recent advancements in ILD biomarker identification include:

- **Fibrosis Biomarkers:** Biomarkers associated with fibrotic activity, such as serum markers (e.g., KL-6, SP-D), extracellular matrix proteins (e.g., MMPs, TIMPs), and molecular signatures (e.g., gene expression profiles), help differentiate fibrotic ILDs from other interstitial lung diseases, monitor disease progression, and predict treatment response in patients with idiopathic pulmonary fibrosis (IPF) and other fibrotic ILDs.
- **Autoimmune Biomarkers:** Biomarkers associated with autoimmune ILDs, such as autoantibodies (e.g., anti-

nuclear antibodies, anti-Jo-1 antibodies), inflammatory cytokines (e.g., TNF-α, IL-6), and immune cell profiles (e.g., lymphocyte subsets), aid in diagnosing specific autoimmune ILDs (e.g., rheumatoid arthritis-associated ILD, systemic sclerosis-associated ILD) and guiding immunomodulatory therapies.

- **Genetic Biomarkers:** Genetic biomarkers, such as telomere length, single nucleotide polymorphisms (SNPs), and gene expression patterns, offer insights into the genetic predisposition, familial clustering, and pathogenic mechanisms underlying ILDs, facilitating early diagnosis, genetic counseling, and targeted therapies in high-risk individuals.

4. Lung Cancer Biomarkers:

Lung cancer is a leading cause of cancer-related mortality worldwide, with diverse molecular subtypes and variable treatment responses. Biomarkers play a pivotal role in lung cancer diagnosis, molecular profiling, and targeted therapy selection. Recent advancements in lung cancer biomarker identification include:

- **Genomic Biomarkers:** Genomic biomarkers, such as EGFR mutations, ALK rearrangements, ROS1 fusions, and BRAF mutations, identify actionable driver mutations in non-small cell lung cancer (NSCLC), guiding targeted therapy selection (e.g., EGFR inhibitors, ALK inhibitors) and improving treatment outcomes in molecularly defined subsets of patients.
- **Liquid Biopsy Biomarkers:** Liquid biopsy biomarkers, including circulating tumor DNA (ctDNA), circulating tumor cells (CTCs), and exosomal RNA, offer non-invasive methods for detecting tumor-specific mutations, monitoring treatment response, and detecting minimal residual disease in lung cancer patients, enabling real-

time disease monitoring and personalized treatment adjustments.
- **Immune Checkpoint Biomarkers:** Immune checkpoint biomarkers, such as PD-L1 expression, tumor mutational burden (TMB), and immune cell infiltrates (e.g., TILs), predict response to immune checkpoint inhibitors (e.g., PD-1/PD-L1 inhibitors) in NSCLC, guiding immunotherapy selection and improving overall survival in patients with advanced or metastatic disease.

Conclusion:

Biomarker identification is at the forefront of respiratory medicine, offering valuable insights into disease pathogenesis, severity, and treatment response across a wide range of respiratory disorders. Recent advancements in biomarker discovery, including inflammatory biomarkers, lung function biomarkers, genetic biomarkers, and liquid biopsy biomarkers, hold promise for improving diagnostic accuracy, guiding treatment decisions, and personalizing therapeutic interventions in asthma, COPD, ILD, and lung cancer. By leveraging these advancements in biomarker identification, healthcare providers can optimize patient care, enhance clinical outcomes, and transform the management of respiratory disorders in the era of precision medicine. Collaborative research efforts, interdisciplinary collaboration, and technology integration are essential for translating biomarker discoveries into clinical practice and improving respiratory health outcomes for individuals worldwide.

Advancements in Gene Therapy and Gene Editing for Respiratory Disorders

Gene therapy and gene editing represent innovative approaches for treating respiratory disorders by targeting underlying genetic defects, modulating gene expression, and correcting aberrant cellular pathways. This section explores recent advancements in gene therapy and gene editing technologies for various respiratory conditions, including cystic fibrosis (CF), alpha-1 antitrypsin deficiency (AATD), primary ciliary dyskinesia (PCD), and genetic lung cancers, highlighting promising strategies, challenges, and future directions in the field.

1. Cystic Fibrosis (CF):

CF is a hereditary disorder caused by mutations in the cystic fibrosis transmembrane conductance regulator (CFTR) gene, leading to impaired chloride ion transport, thickened mucus production, and recurrent pulmonary infections. Gene therapy and gene editing hold promise for treating CF by restoring CFTR function or bypassing defective CFTR channels. Recent advancements in CF gene therapy and gene editing include:

- **Gene Augmentation Therapy:** Gene augmentation therapies, such as adeno-associated virus (AAV) vectors delivering functional CFTR genes, aim to restore CFTR expression in airway epithelial cells, improve chloride ion transport, and reduce mucus viscosity in CF patients, potentially slowing disease progression and improving lung function.
- **Gene Editing Technologies:** Gene editing technologies, such as CRISPR-Cas9, zinc finger nucleases (ZFNs), and transcription activator-like effector nucleases (TALENs), enable precise modification of disease-causing mutations in the CFTR gene, correcting specific genetic defects and restoring CFTR function in patient-derived cells or animal models of CF.
- **Non-Viral Delivery Systems:** Non-viral delivery systems, including lipid nanoparticles, polymer-based

carriers, and cell-penetrating peptides, offer alternative approaches for delivering gene editing tools or CFTR gene constructs to target cells in the airway epithelium, bypassing immune responses and achieving sustained CFTR expression in vivo.

2. Alpha-1 Antitrypsin Deficiency (AATD):

AATD is a genetic disorder characterized by deficient levels of alpha-1 antitrypsin (AAT) protein, leading to unopposed protease activity, tissue destruction, and emphysema. Gene therapy and gene editing hold potential for treating AATD by restoring AAT protein levels or correcting underlying genetic mutations. Recent advancements in AATD gene therapy and gene editing include:

- **AAV-Mediated Gene Delivery:** AAV vectors delivering AAT gene constructs aim to restore physiological levels of AAT protein in the liver, promoting secretion into the bloodstream and protecting the lungs from protease-mediated damage, potentially slowing disease progression and reducing the risk of emphysema in AATD patients.
- **Genome Editing Strategies:** Genome editing strategies, such as CRISPR-Cas9-mediated correction of AAT gene mutations, enable precise modification of disease-causing alleles in patient-derived cells or animal models of AATD, restoring AAT protein expression and function in hepatocytes or lung epithelial cells.
- **Induced Pluripotent Stem Cells (iPSCs):** iPSC-based approaches offer a renewable source of patient-specific cells for disease modeling, drug screening, and gene editing experiments in AATD, providing insights into disease mechanisms, identifying potential therapeutic targets, and developing personalized treatment strategies for individual patients.

3. Primary Ciliary Dyskinesia (PCD):

PCD is a genetic disorder characterized by defective ciliary motility, impaired mucociliary clearance, and recurrent respiratory infections. Gene therapy and gene editing hold promise for treating PCD by restoring ciliary function or correcting underlying genetic mutations. Recent advancements in PCD gene therapy and gene editing include:

- **AAV-Mediated Gene Delivery:** AAV vectors delivering wild-type genes encoding ciliary proteins aim to restore ciliary motility and mucociliary clearance in airway epithelial cells of PCD patients, reducing the frequency and severity of respiratory infections and improving lung function over time.
- **CRISPR-Based Genome Editing:** CRISPR-based genome editing technologies enable precise correction of genetic mutations in PCD-associated genes, such as DNAH5, DNAH11, and CCDC39/CCDC40, restoring ciliary structure and function in patient-derived cells or animal models of PCD, potentially reversing disease phenotypes and improving respiratory health outcomes.
- **Small Molecule Therapies:** Small molecule therapies targeting ciliary assembly, motility, or signaling pathways offer complementary approaches for treating PCD by modulating cellular processes involved in ciliogenesis, ciliary beating, and mucociliary clearance, enhancing the efficacy of gene therapy or gene editing interventions in PCD.

4. Genetic Lung Cancers:

Genetic alterations play a critical role in the development, progression, and treatment response of lung cancers, including driver mutations in oncogenes (e.g., EGFR, ALK, ROS1) and tumor suppressor genes (e.g., TP53, STK11, KEAP1). Gene therapy and gene editing hold promise for targeting specific genetic mutations or dysregulated signaling pathways in lung cancer cells. Recent advancements in genetic lung cancer therapies include:

- **Targeted Gene Delivery:** Targeted gene delivery approaches, such as viral vectors or nanoparticles carrying therapeutic genes or RNA interference (RNAi) molecules, aim to selectively deliver tumor suppressor genes, apoptosis-inducing genes, or siRNAs targeting oncogenic mutations to lung cancer cells, inhibiting tumor growth and metastasis while sparing normal tissues.
- **Genome Editing Strategies:** Genome editing strategies, such as CRISPR-Cas9-mediated disruption of oncogenic driver mutations or precise correction of tumor suppressor gene defects, enable targeted modification of cancer-associated genes in lung cancer cells, inhibiting tumor proliferation, enhancing chemotherapy sensitivity, and overcoming drug resistance mechanisms.
- **Immunogene Therapy:** Immunogene therapy approaches, such as chimeric antigen receptor (CAR) T cell therapy or viral vectors encoding tumor antigens or immune checkpoint inhibitors, aim to enhance anti-tumor immune responses, activate cytotoxic T cells, and overcome immunosuppressive tumor microenvironments in lung cancer, leading to durable tumor regression and long-term remission in select patients.

Conclusion:

Gene therapy and gene editing hold tremendous promise for revolutionizing the treatment of respiratory disorders by targeting underlying genetic defects, modulating gene expression, and correcting aberrant cellular pathways. Recent advancements in gene therapy and gene editing technologies, including AAV-mediated gene delivery, CRISPR-based genome editing, and targeted gene therapies, offer innovative approaches for treating cystic fibrosis, alpha-1 antitrypsin deficiency, primary ciliary dyskinesia, and genetic lung cancers. By leveraging these advancements, healthcare providers can optimize patient care, improve treatment outcomes, and pave the way for personalized precision medicine in respiratory disorders. Collaborative research efforts, interdisciplinary collaboration, and regulatory oversight are essential for translating gene therapy and gene editing innovations into clinical practice and realizing the full potential of these transformative technologies in respiratory medicine.

CHAPTER 8: HOLISTIC APPROACH TO COUGH-VARIANT ASTHMA MANAGEMENT

Exploring Nutritional Considerations in Respiratory Health

Nutrition plays a crucial role in maintaining respiratory health, influencing lung function, immune response, and susceptibility to respiratory diseases. This section delves into the intricate relationship between nutrition and respiratory health, discussing key dietary factors, nutritional interventions, and their impact on various respiratory conditions, including asthma, chronic obstructive pulmonary disease (COPD), cystic fibrosis (CF), and lung cancer.

1. Dietary Factors Influencing Respiratory Health:

Several dietary factors contribute to respiratory health, influencing inflammation, oxidative stress, and immune function in the respiratory system. Key dietary components include:

- **Antioxidants:** Antioxidant-rich foods, such as fruits, vegetables, nuts, and seeds, provide essential vitamins (e.g., vitamin C, vitamin E) and phytochemicals (e.g., flavonoids, carotenoids) that scavenge free radicals, mitigate oxidative stress, and protect against airway inflammation in respiratory diseases.
- **Omega-3 Fatty Acids:** Omega-3 fatty acids, found in fatty fish (e.g., salmon, mackerel), flaxseeds, chia seeds, and walnuts, possess anti-inflammatory properties, modulating inflammatory pathways, and reducing airway inflammation in asthma, COPD, and other respiratory conditions.
- **Vitamin D:** Vitamin D, obtained from sunlight exposure, fortified foods, and supplements, plays a crucial role in immune regulation, enhancing antimicrobial defense mechanisms, and reducing the risk of respiratory infections, asthma exacerbations, and COPD exacerbations.
- **Magnesium:** Magnesium-rich foods, such as leafy greens, legumes, nuts, and whole grains, contribute to bronchodilation, muscle relaxation, and airflow regulation in the respiratory tract, improving lung function and symptom control in asthma and COPD.

2. Nutritional Interventions in Respiratory Diseases:

Nutritional interventions play a vital role in managing respiratory diseases, optimizing lung function, and enhancing quality of life for patients. Key nutritional interventions include:

- **Balanced Diet:** Adopting a balanced diet rich in fruits, vegetables, whole grains, lean proteins, and healthy fats provides essential nutrients, vitamins, and minerals necessary for optimal respiratory health, immune function, and disease prevention.

- **Weight Management:** Maintaining a healthy body weight through proper nutrition and regular physical activity is essential for preventing obesity-related respiratory conditions, such as obesity hypoventilation syndrome (OHS), obstructive sleep apnea (OSA), and obesity-related asthma.
- **Nutritional Supplements:** Nutritional supplements, such as vitamin D, omega-3 fatty acids, probiotics, and antioxidant-rich formulations, may be beneficial as adjunctive therapies in respiratory diseases, improving symptom control, reducing exacerbations, and enhancing overall well-being.
- **Hydration:** Adequate hydration is crucial for maintaining airway hydration, mucus clearance, and respiratory function, particularly in individuals with cystic fibrosis, bronchiectasis, or chronic respiratory infections, where thickened mucus can impair lung function and increase susceptibility to respiratory infections.

3. Nutritional Considerations in Specific Respiratory Conditions:

Nutritional considerations vary across different respiratory conditions, reflecting unique pathophysiological mechanisms, nutritional requirements, and therapeutic goals. Key considerations include:

- **Asthma:** In asthma, dietary factors such as allergenic foods, sulfites, and food additives may trigger exacerbations in susceptible individuals, highlighting the importance of dietary assessment, allergen avoidance, and personalized dietary recommendations to minimize asthma symptoms and optimize lung function.
- **COPD:** In COPD, malnutrition, muscle wasting, and cachexia are common complications, necessitating

nutritional support, energy-dense foods, and protein supplementation to maintain muscle mass, improve exercise tolerance, and prevent disease-related complications, such as respiratory infections and hospitalizations.
- **Cystic Fibrosis:** In cystic fibrosis, pancreatic insufficiency, malabsorption, and fat-soluble vitamin deficiencies are prevalent, requiring pancreatic enzyme replacement therapy (PERT), fat-soluble vitamin supplements (A, D, E, K), and high-calorie, high-fat diets to optimize nutrient absorption, growth, and respiratory function in CF patients.
- **Lung Cancer:** In lung cancer, nutritional support plays a critical role in managing cancer-related cachexia, maintaining nutritional status during chemotherapy or radiation therapy, and supporting immune function and treatment tolerance in patients undergoing cancer treatment.

4. Future Directions and Challenges:

Despite significant advancements in understanding the role of nutrition in respiratory health, several challenges and future directions remain:

- **Personalized Nutrition:** Personalized nutrition approaches tailored to individual patient needs, genetic factors, and disease phenotypes hold promise for optimizing respiratory health outcomes and improving treatment efficacy in respiratory diseases.
- **Nutritional Education:** Enhancing nutritional education, counseling, and support for patients with respiratory diseases, caregivers, and healthcare providers is essential for promoting healthy dietary habits, optimizing nutrient intake, and preventing nutritional deficiencies in vulnerable populations.

- **Research and Innovation:** Continued research and innovation in nutritional science, dietary interventions, and nutritional biomarkers are needed to elucidate the mechanistic links between nutrition and respiratory health, identify novel therapeutic targets, and develop evidence-based nutritional strategies for respiratory diseases.

Conclusion:

Nutrition plays a fundamental role in maintaining respiratory health, influencing inflammation, oxidative stress, and immune function in the respiratory system. By understanding the complex interplay between dietary factors, nutritional interventions, and respiratory diseases, healthcare providers can optimize patient care, enhance treatment outcomes, and improve quality of life for individuals with respiratory disorders. Collaborative efforts, interdisciplinary research, and patient-centered approaches are essential for integrating nutritional considerations into respiratory medicine and promoting holistic approaches to respiratory health and well-being.

The Role of Exercise and Physical Activity in Respiratory Health

Exercise and physical activity are integral components of respiratory health, influencing lung function, respiratory muscle strength, and overall well-being. This section explores the multifaceted relationship between exercise, physical activity, and respiratory health, discussing the physiological benefits, therapeutic interventions, and practical considerations for individuals with respiratory conditions, including asthma, chronic obstructive pulmonary disease (COPD), cystic fibrosis

(CF), and lung cancer.

1. Physiological Benefits of Exercise on Respiratory Health:

Regular exercise and physical activity offer numerous physiological benefits for respiratory health, including:

- **Improved Lung Function:** Aerobic exercise enhances pulmonary ventilation, gas exchange, and lung compliance, improving lung function parameters such as forced expiratory volume in one second (FEV1), vital capacity (VC), and peak expiratory flow rate (PEFR) in healthy individuals and those with respiratory conditions.
- **Enhanced Respiratory Muscle Strength:** Exercise training strengthens respiratory muscles, including the diaphragm, intercostals, and accessory muscles, improving respiratory muscle endurance, efficiency, and fatigue resistance, which is particularly beneficial for individuals with COPD, CF, and neuromuscular respiratory disorders.
- **Increased Cardiorespiratory Fitness:** Regular exercise improves cardiorespiratory fitness, aerobic capacity, and exercise tolerance, enhancing oxygen delivery, utilization, and energy metabolism in skeletal muscles, which is essential for optimizing physical performance and daily activities in individuals with respiratory diseases.
- **Reduced Dyspnea and Fatigue:** Exercise training reduces dyspnea (shortness of breath) and fatigue in individuals with respiratory conditions, improving symptom control, functional capacity, and quality of life, while also reducing the risk of exacerbations, hospitalizations, and mortality.

2. Therapeutic Interventions and Exercise Programs:

Exercise-based interventions and pulmonary rehabilitation programs play a crucial role in managing respiratory diseases, optimizing physical function, and improving quality of life for patients. Key components of pulmonary rehabilitation programs include:

- **Exercise Prescription:** Individualized exercise prescriptions tailored to patients' functional capacity, fitness level, and disease severity, incorporating aerobic exercise (e.g., walking, cycling), resistance training, flexibility exercises, and respiratory muscle training, based on comprehensive assessments and patient goals.
- **Educational Components:** Educational components focusing on disease management, medication adherence, breathing techniques, energy conservation strategies, and lifestyle modifications, empowering patients to self-manage their respiratory condition, reduce exacerbations, and achieve optimal health outcomes.
- **Psychosocial Support:** Psychosocial support services, including counseling, stress management, social support networks, and behavioral interventions, address psychological distress, anxiety, depression, and psychosocial barriers to exercise participation, enhancing adherence and engagement in pulmonary rehabilitation programs.
- **Home-Based Exercise Programs:** Home-based exercise programs offer alternative options for patients unable to attend traditional pulmonary rehabilitation centers due to geographical barriers, transportation limitations, or personal preferences, providing personalized exercise regimens, remote monitoring, and telehealth support to optimize adherence and outcomes.

3. Practical Considerations for Exercise and Physical Activity:

Several practical considerations should be taken into account when implementing exercise and physical activity programs for individuals with respiratory conditions:

- **Gradual Progression:** Exercise programs should be initiated at an appropriate intensity and duration, gradually progressing over time to avoid excessive exertion, fatigue, or musculoskeletal injury, particularly in deconditioned individuals or those with exercise intolerance.
- **Monitoring and Evaluation:** Regular monitoring and evaluation of exercise tolerance, symptoms, functional capacity, and patient-reported outcomes are essential for assessing progress, adjusting exercise prescriptions, and optimizing outcomes in pulmonary rehabilitation programs.
- **Adherence and Motivation:** Strategies to enhance exercise adherence and motivation include setting realistic goals, providing positive reinforcement, social support, and feedback, addressing barriers to participation, and fostering a supportive and inclusive exercise environment for patients.
- **Safety Precautions:** Safety precautions, such as pre-exercise screening, medical clearance, monitoring vital signs, and implementing emergency protocols, are essential for ensuring the safety and well-being of participants during exercise sessions, particularly in high-risk populations or individuals with comorbidities.

Conclusion:

Exercise and physical activity play a pivotal role in promoting respiratory health, improving lung function, respiratory muscle strength, and quality of life for individuals with respiratory conditions. By incorporating exercise-based interventions, pulmonary rehabilitation programs, and practical considerations into clinical practice, healthcare providers can optimize patient care, enhance treatment outcomes, and empower individuals to manage their respiratory condition effectively. Collaborative efforts, interdisciplinary collaboration, and patient-centered approaches are essential for integrating exercise and physical activity into respiratory medicine and promoting holistic approaches to respiratory health and well-being.

The Significance of Stress Reduction Techniques in Respiratory Health

Stress reduction techniques play a pivotal role in managing respiratory conditions by mitigating the impact of psychological stress on respiratory symptoms, inflammation, and immune function. This section delves into the importance of stress reduction techniques in respiratory health, exploring their physiological effects, therapeutic benefits, and practical applications in various respiratory disorders, including asthma, chronic obstructive pulmonary disease (COPD), cystic fibrosis (CF), and lung cancer.

1. Physiological Effects of Stress on Respiratory Health:

Psychological stress exerts profound physiological effects on the respiratory system, triggering neuroendocrine responses, autonomic nervous system activation, and immune dysregulation, which can exacerbate respiratory symptoms, inflammation, and airway hyperresponsiveness. Key mechanisms linking stress to respiratory health include:

- **Sympathetic Activation:** Stress activates the sympathetic nervous system, releasing catecholamines (e.g., adrenaline, noradrenaline) and inducing

bronchodilation, tachycardia, and increased airway resistance, exacerbating asthma symptoms and bronchoconstriction.
- **Hypothalamic-Pituitary-Adrenal (HPA) Axis Activation:** Stress stimulates the HPA axis, leading to the release of cortisol and other stress hormones, which modulate immune function, inflammation, and airway reactivity, contributing to asthma exacerbations and COPD flare-ups.
- **Inflammatory Responses:** Chronic stress promotes systemic inflammation, oxidative stress, and immune dysregulation, increasing the production of pro-inflammatory cytokines (e.g., IL-6, TNF-α) and exacerbating airway inflammation, mucus production, and tissue remodeling in respiratory diseases.
- **Altered Breathing Patterns:** Emotional stress and anxiety can disrupt breathing patterns, leading to shallow, rapid breathing (hyperventilation), chest tightness, and dyspnea (shortness of breath), exacerbating respiratory symptoms and triggering panic attacks in susceptible individuals.

2. Therapeutic Benefits of Stress Reduction Techniques:

Stress reduction techniques offer therapeutic benefits for respiratory health by modulating stress responses, promoting relaxation, and restoring physiological balance. Key benefits include:

- **Reduced Airway Hyperresponsiveness:** Stress reduction techniques, such as diaphragmatic breathing, progressive muscle relaxation, and guided imagery, promote parasympathetic activation, reducing airway hyperresponsiveness and bronchoconstriction in asthma and COPD.
- **Improved Symptom Control:** Stress management

interventions, including mindfulness-based stress reduction (MBSR), cognitive-behavioral therapy (CBT), and biofeedback, alleviate anxiety, depression, and psychological distress, improving symptom control, medication adherence, and quality of life in individuals with respiratory diseases.

- **Enhanced Immune Function:** Stress reduction techniques enhance immune function, modulating cytokine production, immune cell activity, and inflammation pathways, which may reduce the frequency and severity of respiratory infections, exacerbations, and hospitalizations in susceptible individuals.
- **Enhanced Treatment Response:** Stress reduction techniques complement traditional medical therapies by enhancing treatment response, reducing corticosteroid resistance, and improving lung function outcomes in patients with asthma, COPD, and other respiratory conditions.

3. Practical Applications of Stress Reduction Techniques:

Integrating stress reduction techniques into clinical practice requires a multidisciplinary approach, tailored to individual patient needs, preferences, and disease characteristics. Practical applications include:

- **Mindfulness-Based Interventions:** Mindfulness-based stress reduction (MBSR), mindfulness-based cognitive therapy (MBCT), and mindfulness meditation techniques cultivate present-moment awareness, acceptance, and non-judgmental attention, reducing stress reactivity, anxiety, and rumination in individuals with respiratory diseases.
- **Relaxation Techniques:** Relaxation techniques, such as deep breathing exercises, progressive muscle relaxation

(PMR), guided imagery, and autogenic training, induce a state of deep relaxation, reducing sympathetic arousal, muscle tension, and respiratory distress in patients with asthma, COPD, and anxiety-related breathing disorders.
- **Cognitive-Behavioral Therapy (CBT):** CBT interventions target maladaptive thought patterns, cognitive distortions, and fear avoidance behaviors associated with respiratory symptoms, empowering patients to challenge negative beliefs, develop coping strategies, and reframe their perceptions of stress and illness in a more adaptive manner.
- **Physical Activity and Exercise:** Regular physical activity and exercise promote stress reduction through the release of endorphins, improvement of mood, and distraction from negative thoughts, enhancing psychological well-being, self-efficacy, and resilience in individuals with respiratory conditions.

4. Future Directions and Challenges:

Despite the therapeutic potential of stress reduction techniques in respiratory health, several challenges and future directions remain:

- **Integration into Clinical Practice:** Integrating stress reduction techniques into routine clinical care requires training, resources, and collaboration between healthcare providers, psychologists, and respiratory therapists to ensure accessibility, effectiveness, and sustainability of interventions.
- **Patient Adherence and Engagement:** Enhancing patient adherence and engagement in stress reduction programs requires addressing barriers such as time constraints, financial limitations, and cultural factors, while also providing education, support, and reinforcement to promote long-term behavior change.

- **Personalized Approaches:** Tailoring stress reduction interventions to individual patient preferences, personality traits, and coping styles enhances relevance, acceptability, and efficacy, recognizing the heterogeneity of stress responses and psychological needs in respiratory diseases.
- **Research and Evaluation:** Continued research and evaluation of stress reduction techniques, including randomized controlled trials, longitudinal studies, and qualitative research, are needed to elucidate their mechanisms of action, optimize intervention protocols, and assess long-term outcomes in diverse populations with respiratory conditions.

Conclusion:

Stress reduction techniques play a critical role in managing respiratory conditions by modulating stress responses, promoting relaxation, and improving psychological well-being for individuals with asthma, COPD, cystic fibrosis, and lung cancer. By incorporating stress reduction interventions into clinical practice, healthcare providers can optimize patient care, enhance treatment outcomes, and promote holistic approaches to respiratory health and well-being. Collaborative efforts, interdisciplinary collaboration, and patient-centered approaches are essential for integrating stress reduction techniques into respiratory medicine and addressing the psychological dimensions of respiratory diseases.

The Importance of Sleep Hygiene in Respiratory Health

Sleep hygiene encompasses a set of practices and habits aimed at promoting restful and quality sleep. Its significance in respiratory health lies in its potential to improve symptoms, enhance immune function, and optimize overall well-being. This section explores the role of sleep hygiene in respiratory health, highlighting its physiological effects, therapeutic benefits, and practical applications in managing various respiratory conditions, including asthma, chronic obstructive pulmonary disease (COPD), cystic fibrosis (CF), and sleep-disordered breathing.

1. Physiological Effects of Sleep on Respiratory Health:

Sleep plays a vital role in maintaining respiratory health, facilitating cellular repair, immune function, and metabolic homeostasis. Key physiological effects of sleep on respiratory health include:

- **Respiratory Muscle Relaxation:** During sleep, respiratory muscle tone decreases, and airway resistance increases, leading to a reduction in airflow and ventilation, particularly during non-rapid eye movement (NREM) sleep stages, which may exacerbate airway obstruction in individuals with obstructive respiratory disorders.
- **Airway Patency:** Sleep influences upper airway dynamics, tone, and collapsibility, predisposing susceptible individuals to airway collapse, snoring, and obstructive sleep apnea (OSA), which can lead to intermittent hypoxemia, hypercapnia, and disrupted sleep architecture, impairing respiratory function and exacerbating respiratory symptoms.
- **Immune Regulation:** Sleep modulates immune function, inflammation, and cytokine production, enhancing host defense mechanisms, promoting tissue repair, and regulating inflammatory pathways, which may reduce susceptibility to respiratory infections and exacerbations in individuals with respiratory diseases.
- **Gas Exchange:** Sleep influences gas exchange,

oxygenation, and carbon dioxide elimination, with alterations in breathing patterns, respiratory rate, and tidal volume during different sleep stages, affecting arterial blood gases, pH balance, and respiratory drive in individuals with respiratory conditions.

2. Therapeutic Benefits of Sleep Hygiene Practices:

Optimizing sleep hygiene practices offers therapeutic benefits for respiratory health by promoting restorative sleep, enhancing sleep quality, and reducing the risk of sleep-related respiratory disturbances. Key benefits include:

- **Improved Symptom Control:** Adequate sleep hygiene practices, such as maintaining a consistent sleep schedule, optimizing sleep environment, and reducing sleep disruptions, can improve symptom control, reduce nocturnal awakenings, and enhance daytime functioning in individuals with respiratory diseases.
- **Enhanced Immune Function:** Quality sleep promotes immune function, enhancing the body's ability to mount an effective immune response to respiratory pathogens, reducing the risk of respiratory infections, exacerbations, and complications in susceptible individuals, including those with asthma, COPD, and CF.
- **Reduced Daytime Fatigue:** Restful and uninterrupted sleep improves daytime alertness, cognitive function, and psychomotor performance, reducing daytime fatigue, sleepiness, and impairment in individuals with respiratory disorders, enhancing productivity, and quality of life.
- **Optimized Treatment Response:** Adequate sleep hygiene practices complement medical therapies for respiratory conditions by enhancing treatment response, reducing medication requirements, and improving treatment adherence, thereby optimizing disease management and

long-term outcomes.

3. Practical Applications of Sleep Hygiene Practices:

Implementing sleep hygiene practices requires a multidisciplinary approach, tailored to individual patient needs, preferences, and disease characteristics. Practical applications include:

- **Sleep Schedule Regulation:** Maintaining a regular sleep-wake schedule by going to bed and waking up at the same time each day, including weekends, helps regulate the body's internal clock, synchronize circadian rhythms, and promote restorative sleep in individuals with respiratory diseases.
- **Sleep Environment Optimization:** Creating a conducive sleep environment by minimizing noise, light, and temperature disruptions, using comfortable bedding and supportive mattresses, and removing electronic devices or screens from the bedroom promotes relaxation, reduces sleep disturbances, and enhances sleep quality.
- **Stress Reduction Techniques:** Incorporating stress reduction techniques, such as mindfulness meditation, deep breathing exercises, or progressive muscle relaxation, before bedtime helps alleviate anxiety, tension, and arousal, promoting relaxation, and facilitating sleep onset in individuals with respiratory disorders.
- **Limiting Stimulants and Substances:** Avoiding stimulants, such as caffeine, nicotine, and alcohol, close to bedtime, and reducing fluid intake to minimize nocturia (nighttime urination) can prevent sleep disturbances, promote uninterrupted sleep, and improve sleep continuity in individuals with respiratory conditions.

4. Future Directions and Challenges:

Despite the therapeutic potential of sleep hygiene practices in respiratory health, several challenges and future directions remain:

- **Education and Awareness:** Enhancing education and awareness of sleep hygiene practices among healthcare providers, patients, and the general public is essential for promoting adoption, adherence, and sustainability of healthy sleep habits, recognizing sleep as a vital component of respiratory health and overall well-being.
- **Integrating Behavioral Interventions:** Integrating behavioral interventions, such as cognitive-behavioral therapy for insomnia (CBT-I), sleep hygiene education, and sleep restriction therapy, into routine clinical care for respiratory diseases requires training, resources, and collaboration between respiratory specialists, sleep medicine practitioners, and behavioral therapists.
- **Identifying High-Risk Populations:** Identifying high-risk populations for sleep-related respiratory disturbances, such as OSA, nocturnal hypoventilation, or restless leg syndrome, and implementing targeted screening, assessment, and intervention strategies can improve detection rates, facilitate early diagnosis, and prevent complications in vulnerable individuals.
- **Research and Innovation:** Continued research and innovation in sleep medicine, respiratory physiology, and behavioral sleep interventions are needed to elucidate the mechanistic links between sleep and respiratory health, optimize sleep hygiene practices, and develop evidence-based guidelines for managing sleep-related issues in respiratory diseases.

Conclusion:

Sleep hygiene practices play a critical role in maintaining respiratory health, promoting restful and quality sleep, and reducing the risk of sleep-related respiratory disturbances in individuals with respiratory conditions. By incorporating sleep hygiene interventions into clinical practice, healthcare providers can optimize patient care, enhance treatment outcomes, and improve overall well-being. Collaborative efforts, interdisciplinary collaboration, and patient-centered approaches are essential for integrating sleep hygiene practices into respiratory medicine and promoting holistic approaches to respiratory health and sleep wellness.

Exploring Herbal and Alternative Therapies in Respiratory Health

Herbal and alternative therapies have gained popularity as complementary approaches to conventional medical treatments for respiratory conditions. This section delves into the diverse landscape of herbal and alternative therapies, examining their mechanisms of action, therapeutic potential, and evidence-based applications in managing various respiratory disorders, including asthma, chronic obstructive pulmonary disease (COPD), cystic fibrosis (CF), and bronchitis.

1. Mechanisms of Action of Herbal and Alternative Therapies:

Herbal and alternative therapies encompass a wide range of botanicals, dietary supplements, and traditional remedies with diverse mechanisms of action, including:

- **Anti-inflammatory Effects:** Many herbal remedies possess anti-inflammatory properties, inhibiting the production of pro-inflammatory cytokines (e.g., TNF-α, IL-6) and modulating immune responses in

the respiratory tract, which may alleviate airway inflammation and improve symptom control in respiratory diseases.
- **Antioxidant Activity:** Herbal supplements rich in antioxidants, such as flavonoids, polyphenols, and vitamins, scavenge free radicals, reduce oxidative stress, and protect against airway damage, mucosal injury, and respiratory infections associated with respiratory conditions.
- **Bronchodilator Effects:** Certain herbal remedies exhibit bronchodilator effects by relaxing smooth muscle tone, increasing airway diameter, and improving airflow dynamics, which may alleviate bronchoconstriction, dyspnea, and cough in individuals with asthma, COPD, or bronchospastic disorders.
- **Mucolytic and Expectorant Properties:** Herbal therapies with mucolytic and expectorant properties promote mucus clearance, reduce sputum viscosity, and facilitate airway clearance mechanisms, which may alleviate congestion, cough, and respiratory symptoms in individuals with bronchitis or chronic mucus hypersecretion.

2. Therapeutic Potential of Herbal and Alternative Therapies:

Herbal and alternative therapies offer potential therapeutic benefits for respiratory health by addressing symptom management, disease modification, and overall well-being. Key therapeutic potentials include:

- **Symptom Relief:** Herbal remedies may provide symptomatic relief for respiratory symptoms such as cough, wheezing, dyspnea, and chest tightness, offering an alternative or adjunctive approach to conventional pharmacotherapy in individuals with respiratory conditions.

- **Disease Modification:** Some herbal supplements possess disease-modifying properties, modulating underlying pathophysiological processes, such as inflammation, oxidative stress, and airway remodeling, which may slow disease progression, reduce exacerbations, and improve long-term outcomes in respiratory diseases.
- **Improved Quality of Life:** Herbal and alternative therapies may enhance quality of life by alleviating respiratory symptoms, improving physical function, and reducing medication side effects, thereby promoting overall well-being and patient satisfaction in individuals with chronic respiratory conditions.
- **Adjunctive Therapy:** Herbal and alternative therapies can complement conventional medical treatments by addressing specific symptoms, enhancing treatment efficacy, and reducing reliance on pharmacological interventions, particularly in individuals with treatment-resistant or poorly controlled respiratory diseases.

3. Evidence-Based Applications of Herbal and Alternative Therapies:

The evidence base for herbal and alternative therapies in respiratory health varies widely, with some remedies supported by clinical trials and systematic reviews, while others lack robust scientific validation. Evidence-based applications include:

- **Herbal Supplements:** Herbal supplements such as Boswellia serrata, Ginkgo biloba, and Pelargonium sidoides have demonstrated efficacy in improving respiratory symptoms, reducing exacerbations, and enhancing quality of life in individuals with asthma, COPD, or acute respiratory infections, based on clinical trials and meta-analyses.

- **Traditional Remedies:** Traditional remedies such as ginger, honey, and turmeric have been used for centuries in folk medicine to alleviate respiratory symptoms, soothe throat irritation, and enhance immune function, with emerging evidence supporting their therapeutic potential in respiratory conditions.
- **Mind-Body Therapies:** Mind-body therapies such as yoga, tai chi, and qigong incorporate breathing exercises, relaxation techniques, and mindful movement practices, which may improve respiratory function, reduce stress, and enhance overall well-being in individuals with asthma, COPD, or sleep-related breathing disorders.
- **Acupuncture and Acupressure:** Acupuncture and acupressure techniques target specific acupoints along meridian channels, regulating energy flow, and restoring balance in the body, which may alleviate respiratory symptoms, improve lung function, and reduce medication use in individuals with asthma or COPD.

4. Practical Considerations and Safety Concerns:

Despite their potential benefits, herbal and alternative therapies pose practical considerations and safety concerns for individuals with respiratory conditions:

- **Standardization and Quality Control:** Herbal supplements lack standardized formulations, potency, and quality control measures, raising concerns about variability, contamination, and adverse effects, emphasizing the importance of using reputable brands and seeking guidance from healthcare providers.
- **Drug Interactions:** Herbal remedies may interact with conventional medications, affecting drug metabolism, absorption, or efficacy, which can pose risks for individuals with respiratory conditions, particularly those on multiple medications or with comorbidities,

necessitating caution and close monitoring.
- **Allergic Reactions:** Some herbal supplements, botanical extracts, or traditional remedies may trigger allergic reactions, sensitivities, or adverse effects in susceptible individuals, highlighting the importance of allergy testing, patch testing, or cautious use in individuals with known allergies or sensitivities.
- **Regulatory Oversight:** Herbal and alternative therapies are subject to limited regulatory oversight, quality assurance, and evidence-based scrutiny compared to pharmaceutical drugs, necessitating informed decision-making, consumer awareness, and transparency in product labeling and marketing.

Conclusion:

Herbal and alternative therapies offer potential therapeutic benefits for respiratory health by addressing symptom management, disease modification, and overall well-being in individuals with respiratory conditions. By integrating evidence-based herbal remedies, traditional therapies, and complementary approaches into clinical practice, healthcare providers can offer personalized, holistic care, and empower patients to explore safe and effective options for managing their respiratory health. Collaborative efforts, interdisciplinary research, and patient-centered approaches are essential for advancing our understanding of herbal and alternative therapies in respiratory medicine and promoting integrative approaches to respiratory health and wellness.

Printed in Great Britain
by Amazon